beautiful
you

a daily guide to Radical Self-Acceptance

rosie molinary

SEAL

Beautiful You

A Daily Guide to Radical Self-Acceptance

Copyright ©2010 by Rosie Molinary

Published by

SEAL PRESS

A Member of the Perseus Books Group

1700 Fourth Street | Berkeley, California

Library of Congress Cataloging-in-Publication Data

Molinary, Rosie.

  Beautiful you : a daily guide to radical self-acceptance / Rosie Molinary.

     p. cm.

  ISBN 978-1-58005-331-0

  1. Self-perception. 2. Mind and body. 3. Self-consciousness (Awareness) I. Title.

  BF697.5.S43M65 2010

  155.3'33—dc22

                    2010014823

9 8 7 6 5 4 3 2

Cover and interior design by Kate Basart/Union Pageworks

Printed in the United States of America

Distributed by Publishers Group West

To the hijas and m'ijas of Circle de Luz,
because your beauty inspires and your brilliance illuminates.

Contents

Introduction

At eight years old, my best friend, Jenny, and I conspired to get rid of our fat. It was 1981. We were entering the second grade. We barely watched television, so we had no real idea of media-generated ideals. And yet, we thought we were fat. Years later I would see pictures of us, as if for the first time, and realize that we were actually lean and willowy.

At eighteen, I arrived at college to find that I looked like no one else. My self-consciousness was amplified when a friend suggested that I try highlights on my black curls. In that moment, I internalized the idea that my hair wasn't right, that I wasn't right.

At twenty-four, I was a high school teacher, telling my students they were brilliant and smart and could do anything. Some days, despite my earnest efforts, I couldn't make them buy the truth I was selling. I packed healthy lunches every day for one of my soccer players who wouldn't feed herself. When another one of my athletes regularly broke into so much anger that no one could escape her derision, not even herself, I would sweep her into my arms and hold her, trying to calm her into believing in her own worth. When one of my mentees in a summer program said her boyfriend wanted sex, I reminded her that what she wanted was just as important. When the last day of school came, I called my students, one by one, to the front of the classroom while I played a song that reminded me of him or her—"Closer to Fine" by the Indigo Girls, "Pride" by U2, "Everything Is Everything" by Lauryn Hill, or "A Wink and a Smile" by Harry Connick Jr.—and a reverent silence fell over that space, my students basking in being acknowledged. Each would sit on a stool in the front of the room while I celebrated a trait I appreciated most about him or her— inquisitiveness, compassion, passion, wisdom, patience—and my students relished the fact that their brilliance was being recognized.

At thirty-four, I was having lunch with nine seventh-grade girls at a local middle school when one of the guidance counselors, a woman in her late fifties whom I knew and admired, walked in to say hello. It was school picture day, and each girl had taken great care to get ready that morning.

"Are you getting your picture taken?" one girl asked the counselor.

"I hate having my picture taken," she answered. "When I was in fourth grade, I was the tallest kid in school. When I went to pose for my school picture, the photographer, who was a man, screamed, 'We have a big one here!' I've hated being photographed ever since."

"Do you like your height now?" I asked.

For a moment she looked confused.

"I love my height," she said. "And I shouldn't mind having my picture taken anymore. I have given that man so much power over my life, and he's probably not even alive anymore."

I know what it is like to want to believe in yourself wholeheartedly only to have episodes in your life lead you to question your own beauty and radiance. I know what it is like to try to help someone galvanize her own power, realize her own brilliance. It is, what I most wish to offer—whether I am spending time with a little girl in my life, a dear friend, an acquaintance, or one of my students. And it is what is offered here, in *Beautiful You: A Daily Guide to Radical Self-Acceptance*.

In this book, you will find down-to-earth advice on how you can realize your own brilliance every day. But the true value of the book does not come from what's written on its pages. It comes from doing the work, from journeying toward insight and action through the exercises and reflections. It is a tool kit for self-awareness, positive self-esteem, and a healthy body image. The magic of this book begins with your intention—your desire to tackle what is limiting you, and your decision to love yourself, be happy, and feel satisfied with your body.

A poor body image isn't usually at the root of a woman's negative feelings about herself. A poor self-concept and lack of confidence are often at the core of a negative body image. Having a negative self-image or a negative body image is like always having a gate-crashing critic watching the events of your life as they unfold. What I have found over time is that self-acceptance is what most dynamically changes our negative self-concept and body image. And you can only find self-acceptance through the hard but meaningful work of assessing where you are, seeing where you have been, and planning where you are going—while enhancing your life along the way.

This book will take you on a journey that encourages you to develop a clearer sense of yourself. Over time, once you have a clearer sense of self, self-confidence will become a habit. Confidence is born from proof, and proof of your worth comes when you have cultivated and embraced your whole self. A positive self-esteem comes with knowing your truth, your reality, and arriving at a self-mastery that allows for resilience, pro-activity, and brilliance. And while this book's journey might begin by taking you more deeply inward, in the end it will help you move beyond yourself and into the world, where acting on what you have to offer does so much more good than worrying about what you look like.

The secret to success with *Beautiful You* is completing its guided daily practices. Daily practices yield new patterns of thinking, and those patterns ultimately yield new habits that will renew your sense of self in a positive, dynamic, healthy way. This book quiets you and moves you to find clarity; it encourages you to develop your own insights through compassionate observation and careful execution. This is a book that will leave you unsettled at times, so that you can eventually become more settled in life; a book that challenges you at times, so that you can develop a fresh outlook. By giving you the opportunity to consider, observe, do, and be, this book will help you recognize what is really beautiful—you, as you are. You are being invited to begin a process that will yield self-knowledge and deliver self-mastery.

We can all grow, no matter our history. We can all recognize our brilliance. Recognizing beauty, as it turns out, is a choice. You can see it the way the world hands it to you, or you can see it the way you want to see it.

How to Use This Book

For some of you, this will be a first attempt at trying to understand and positively influence your self-concept. What *Beautiful You* offers to every reader are the tools to understand and overcome any dissatisfaction you might have with yourself, and to magnify what makes you brilliant. This book offers you the resources you'll need to form a better vision of yourself, a process for following through, and company for the journey. The supplies you will need for the journey are easy to acquire: A favorite pen and a personal journal, referred throughout the book as your *Beautiful You* journal, are essential.

There are a number of ways to use this book. I encourage you to use it in the way that makes the most sense for you. Some of you will begin on Day 1 and read the chapters in order, to Day 365. Others may check the Table of Contents and start by reading about specific topics that speak to them. You can work through the book alone or in a group. No matter how you enter it, the journey will be rich, and it will lead you to find something very important: yourself.

Feel free to begin by surveying the pages to get a sense of how the book progresses over the course of a year. Don't worry about spoiling the ending. This is a book that you *do,* not just read, so perusing it won't take away the surprise, joy, or revelations to come.

Each daily practice begins with a passage that may be part autobiographical, part informational, part inspirational, and ends with a suggested task for the day. I encourage you not to feel overwhelmed by the tasks. Many of them are short. Some are more fun than tedious. All of them are a gift to yourself and your world.

Choose a time each day to read the passage and plan for how or when you will do the exercise of the day. Some readers may find that it makes sense to read each passage with a morning cup of tea or coffee. Others may choose to read a passage each night. If the task involves a journal exercise or other reflection, you can do it right then. If the exercise requires you to take some sort of action, to step out in your world, you can save it for the next day.

Some passages and tasks will really appeal to you; others may turn you off. Resist the urge to turn away from the ones that seem daunting. Those are often the exercises you need most. There are some tasks that just won't be relevant to you, given where you are in your life. If that's the case, just move on. Finally, you will discover that some of these tasks—looking up when you are walking, eating mindfully, quieting your critic—can be done every day. Ultimately, each task is designed to be practiced at least once, but I hope you find that many of the tasks become part of your routine—that completing them that day is really only the beginning of your journey with them.

This book was written as a guide to an individual's journey, but by no means do you need to make the journey alone. In fact, doing it in partnership with someone else or in a group may even push you to engage more deeply in the process. If you'd like to do it in a dyad or group, here is some insight on how to facilitate the process.

First, how do you find your dyad or group? Consider the people you feel closest to. The greatest support and encouragement will come from those who believe in you. Keep the group to a reasonable size so that everyone will have the opportunity to participate.

Before you begin the exercises together you can each share your intention for engaging in the process. Also share your hesitations, worries, and hopes. Then, as a group or a partnership, discuss your shared goal. It can be more than encouraging one another on your journeys. Share your visions. Lay it all out on the table. Then consider some guidelines for the process. Your first guidelines might reflect how you wish to interact with each other as you share and encourage.

Here are a few guidelines that should be a part of your list.

Our brilliance shines most when we are in a place where we know that we are both accepted and safe. Our space and time together will be one that fosters both qualities.

Everything shared is held sacred and in confidence. Our journey is our individual story to tell. No one else should share someone else's story outside of the group without expressed permission.

Our feedback will always be honest, thoughtful, and supportive and will build on our strengths.

Our goal is always to grow and move forward. We will support one another in this process and push one another to recognize, celebrate, and offer her brilliance to the world.

You will also want to consider when and how you will come together. For some groups, it might make sense to have a monthly meet-up where you discuss the exercises that have had the most impact for you. It might also make sense to have a weekly check-in over email.

Mothers may choose to take this journey with their daughters. If you are completing *Beautiful You* with a teenage or young adult daughter, it might be helpful for you to read ahead every Sunday to see what is coming and to determine how you'd like to navigate the exercises and your sharing based on any familial history.

Helpful questions along the way for every dyad, cluster, and group to consider in their regular meetings include:

How are you doing?

What is challenging you about this process?

What is satisfying to you about this process?

How have you grown?

What have you learned?

What has changed?

What are you noticing?

What did you love doing?

What did you skip and why?

What are you anticipating?

What was an epiphany you had this month?

I wish I could promise you that your path on this journey will always be up a ladder, that you will climb past an issue and never revisit it again. But that is not the nature of our lives. Instead, our journeys are more cyclical. Like the lover who comes back at different times in our life, so will some of our issues. Our greatest hope is that when we see the old lover again, when the old issues resurface, we can approach them as the person we are today, not as the person we were the last time we dealt with them.

Here is what I want for each of us: the ability to experience the world as we see ourselves, not as how others see us or how we perceive we are seen; the ability to live now rather than someday. I want us to understand that a negative self-image is a beacon, calling us to explore what is really going on deep within. I want us to use that beacon to arrive at a place of understanding and clarity. I want each of us to break free from the idea that narrowly defined external beauty is everything, and instead embrace and see the beauty in our inner selves. By taking the *Beautiful You* journey, you alight on a path that will be good to you, that will allow you to settle into who you are, that will give you the tools you need to be your truest self.

There will be days when you want to turn away from this journey, when it will feel too long, too demanding, too difficult. The important things in life are hard that way; the tough things teach us who we are, the impossible things allow us to arrive at what matters. There is no quick fix to improving our sense of selves. Every day, you can find a story of someone who medicated herself with plastic surgery, weight loss programs, or new relationships in order to find happiness, only to find that she's not that happy with the very thing that she thought would cure her.

There is no quick fix to improving your self-concept. This book guides you through the slow, deliberate process of enhancing your life through your own personal empowerment. Give yourself the room and time and attention to grow your sense of self. However you feel about yourself, those feelings were not created in just one day—and addressing how you feel about yourself will also take more than a day, and more than several. Changing your self-image takes time, attention, discipline, and desire. And it gives us back so much more than that.

Please be aware that this book is no substitute for therapy or treatment if you are suffering from an eating disorder or body dysmorphic disorder. If you suspect that your problems may be clinical in nature, I encourage you to get the help you need from a trained professional as the first step in your journey.

Poor self-image is not just the province of the young. It affects women of all ages and is not limited to any socioeconomic situation, race, culture, or worldview. The way we feel about our bodies, our dissatisfaction with our bodies, doesn't exist in a vacuum. It bleeds out, affecting how we feel about ourselves and the life we are living.

Too often, we believe we will finally be content when our body changes in some way. Actually, we'll be content only when our mind changes, when we give ourselves permission and the tools to be content. The key to feeling better isn't looking better. It is feeling better about our lives and better understanding what our bodies really are–vehicles in which we can experience life. Our bodies are not life itself; they are objects of motion, not admiration.

If we stop the world's racket and engage deliberately in our lives, we change ourselves. *Beautiful You* provides the tools–vision, passion, purpose, resilience, productivity–for every woman who wants to see beauty in a way that is true to who she is and not in the way the world hands it to her.

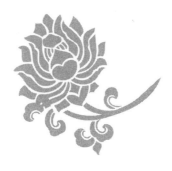

DAY

— 1 —

Begin

The book that captivated my heart and mind as a child was *Harriet the Spy*. Harriet ignited the curiosity in me, as well as my inner writer. But Harriet actually ignited something else. She ignited the seeker and the discoverer in me, and those parts of my personality are, ultimately, what led me on my journey to find myself. Soon after reading about Harriet's many notebooks, I began keeping my own stream-of-consciousness journals filled with bad poetry, dramatic musings, and hyperbolic dreams. By the time I reached high school, journaling was my lifeline. My journals were where I confided what I was feeling, how I was dealing with things, what I was planning. I also found that my journals kept me honest. It was outside my character to write one thing and do another. So what I wrote, I did.

Through journaling, I had the opportunity to get to know myself at a relatively young age. Many people, especially teens, live on the surface, operating at breakneck speeds and never exploring the depths within them. We're too busy to listen to what is going on inside of us because we are manipulating, reacting, adjusting to the world outside of us. To really know my self, my stories, and my voice, I had to have silence, an entryway, a slowing down. Journaling provided me that and more.

With journaling, you see the patterns of your life; you claim—or reclaim—who you really are; you coach yourself into becoming the someone you imagined; you arrive at a sense of balance, of yourself, of wholeness. You can discover productive patterns and nonproductive patterns in your life, and you can choose to embrace the ones that move you forward. A significant part of the *Beautiful You* experience will be accomplished through journaling. Already, you have purchased a *Beautiful You* journal. You will use it for exercises recommended in each daily practice, but I also encourage you to use it for your own lists, confessional laments, stream-of-consciousness ideas, and dreams. There is no right way to journal. There is only this: the desire to record what you think and feel so that you can become better acquainted with yourself, so that you are better in touch with your own brilliance. The most important thing is that you give yourself time and room to write—and thus, to get to know yourself and grow in the coming year.

Today —— Open your *Beautiful You* journal and consider these questions. What are your hopes—personally and for the world—with regard to body image and beauty perception? How can you begin to live your hopes today? Thinking about what you want most for yourself and for the world allows you to act on that information.

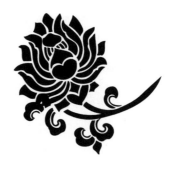

DAY

2

Pledge Allegiance to Yourself

D eciding to be a body champion is the first step on your journey to developing and boosting your self esteem and body image. Thinking through the nuances of such a commitment can help your journey be successful.

Today ⟶ Review and sign this Body Warrior Pledge. In your *Beautiful You* journal, make a note of which statement will take the most determination for you to embrace, why, and how you plan on doing it.

The Body Warrior Pledge ⟶ Because I understand that my love and respect for my body are metaphors of my love and respect for my self and soul, I pledge:

- ◆ To stop berating my body and to begin celebrating the vessel that I have been given. I will remember the amazing things my body has given me: the ability to experience the world with a breadth of senses, the ability to perceive and express love, the ability to comfort and soothe, and the ability to fight, provide, and care for humanity.

- ◆ To understand that my body is an opportunity not a scapegoat.

- ◆ To be the primary source of my confidence. I will not rely on others to define my worth.

- ◆ To let envy dissipate and allow admiration to be a source of compassion by offering compliments to others.

- ◆ To gently but firmly stand up for myself when someone says something harmful.

- To change the inner monologue in my head to one that sees possibility not problems, potential not shortcomings, blessings not imperfections.

- To give my body the things that it needs to do its work well: plenty of water, ample movement, stretches, rest, and good nutrition, and to limit or eliminate the things that do not nurture my body.

- To see exercise as a way to improve my internal health and strength instead of a way to fight or control my body.

- To understand that my weight is not good or bad. It is just a number, and I am only good.

- To love my body and myself today. I do not have to weigh ten pounds less, have longer hair, or have my degree in my hand to have worth. I have worth just as I am, and I embrace that power.

- To recognize my body's strengths.

- To no longer put off the things that I wish to experience because I am waiting to do them in a different body.

- To understand that a body, just like a personality, is like a fingerprint: a wonderful embodiment of my uniqueness.

Signature | Date

— 3 —

Consider How You Feel About Yourself

This *Beautiful You* journey is meant to help you enhance your self-awareness while boosting your self-esteem and sense of body satisfaction. To begin, it is important to know and understand where you have been with regard to these areas, how you got there, and where you would like to go.

Today ——— In your *Beautiful You* journal, answer these questions. How do you feel about yourself? Why is that the case? What will a healthy sense of self and a healthy life give to you?

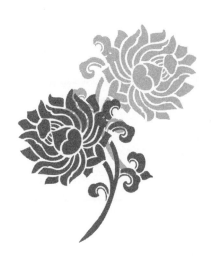

— 4 —

Consider How Body Image Has Impacted Your Life

We can become so embroiled in our personal assessments that we no longer notice the way our sense of self affects our daily life. Yet it often does. Understanding your body image history can be extremely helpful in creating a new landscape for yourself and your future.

Today —— In your *Beautiful You* journal, answer these questions completely. How has body image impacted your daily life and outlook? What have been your challenges and triumphs with body image over time? What have you denied and allowed yourself because of your perception of your appearance? How has your personality changed because of your sense of your appearance? What have you gained or lost because of your body image?

— 5 —

Consider Your Vision

I t is impossible to live the life we want most if we haven't taken time to imagine it. By knowing what it is we want and where we are today in relation to our dreams, we can put ourselves in the position to pursue our possibilities.

Today —— In your *Beautiful You* journal, answer these questions. What is your vision for yourself? What do you wish or want for yourself? How is that different from who you are or where you are today? What do you think would make you feel more confident?

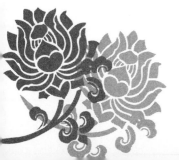

Ditch the Fat Chat

We've all been there. A girlfriend complains about her thighs, and we just can't help but bring up our stomach. Then it becomes a body-hatred free-for-all. A study published in the June 2007 issue of *Body Image: An International Journal of Research* revealed that if a woman criticizes herself, those around her tend to add their own negative self-impressions to the conversation—even if they had just described their body image as "positive" or "high." Sure, there are all sorts of reasons that a woman might do this—to build camaraderie, to be polite—but because those statements might end up having a significant impact on one's self-perception, why not build camaraderie in other ways and stop the personal attacks?

Today —— When a woman criticizes herself in front of you, don't join in. Instead, celebrate what you love about her or tell her just how wrong she is. When you are inclined to begin your own body-bashing, stop yourself. We do ourselves and others a disservice when we allow these critiques to carry on.

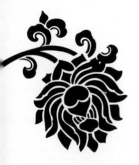

— 7 —

Name Your Inner Critic

Too many of us have that voice inside our head that just nags, nags, nags us about everything. She tells us that we aren't skinny enough, that our hair is bad, that our style sucks, that we are not of value. She exhausts us and extinguishes us and deserves to be put in her place.

Today —— Give that voice a name—Sylvia, for example, or Agnes. And when she pipes up today, put her in her place.

"Agnes, I am not listening to you."

"Sylvia, you are so negative."

And then spin her criticism on its head.

"Agnes, it doesn't matter if I am skinny in your eyes. It matters whether or not I am healthy in mine."

"Sylvia, my hair looks perfectly fine."

Calling out your inner critic and changing her direction is a vital step in moving from negative self-image to positive.

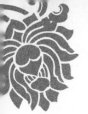

8

Create a Self-Appreciation Jar

When I was touring for my previous book, *Hijas Americanas: Beauty, Body Image, and Growing Up Latina*, I had the pleasure of visiting Amherst, Massachusetts, for several days to speak at the University of Massachusetts Amherst, Amherst College, and Mount Holyoke College. One of the things that I often talk about is the need to modify our own language—what we project about ourselves—and the language of others. When someone says she hates her nose, instead of saying "I hate my cellulite" in order to feel companionship with that person, say, "I can't imagine why you would hate your nose, and you have a smile that lights up the world" (or whatever else might be the case).

After my talk at Amherst College, I met some roommates who told me about a jar they keep in their suite. Anyone who says anything bad about herself has to deposit some cash into the jar. When it adds up to enough for a quality loaf of bread, they hit the bakery. What a novel way to break your self-deprecation habit and to use the times you are mean to yourself as an opportunity to reinvest in yourself. As individuals, we shouldn't normalize our body hatred, letting unkind words pass our lips without a thought. We should catch and correct ourselves because our whole lives are affected by how we think and speak about our bodies.

Today ⟶ You've been ditching the fat chat for a few days. Now let's take it a step further. Find a bowl, vase, or piggy bank to catch your quarters when you knock yourself, and watch your self-awareness soar and your habits change. We can all change our language—and our minds.

Consider What Your Words Are Really Saying

Our words aren't just empty. They are a road map to how we are feeling about ourselves. If we make observations about our language, we can gather essential information that will help us be and do better.

Today ——— As you begin to make Self-Apprecation Jar deposits for things you no longer want to be saying, take note of your words. What is it you say about yourself? Why do you say it? What are your emotions when you say it? Write it down in your *Beautiful You* journal, then consider what you are really saying. If "I am fat" is always coming to your lips, think those words through until you are holding onto some truth. Are you unhappy with your weight because you would like to be more healthy—perhaps able to walk up stairs without losing your breath or get off a certain type of medication—or are you unhappy with your weight because it doesn't meet a Hollywood standard of beauty? By really examining the motivation behind your words, you can see the truth and act accordingly.

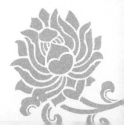

— 10 —

Consider Your Positive Memories

I teach a seminar on body image at the University of North Carolina at Charlotte. In the class, the very first assignment my students face is writing a body image autobiography. I explain to my students that to better interpret, experience, and study how body image is played out in our culture, we must understand some of our own paradigms. Then I ask them to answer twenty questions as honestly as they can, without filtering their thoughts. One part of the exercise looks at their positive memories and what they appreciate about themselves.

Today —— Answer these questions in your *Beautiful You* journal. What do you appreciate most about yourself? What are you most confident about? What is the first positive memory you have of yourself? Was anyone there to witness that moment? If so, who was there and how did he, she, or they react?

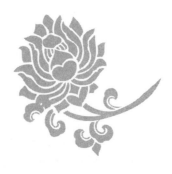

— 11 —

Realize That You Are Not Your Body

Growing up, there were times when I struggled with what my looks and ethnicity meant. It wasn't that I had a difficult time assessing myself; it was more about how overwhelmed I felt with how other people interpreted my looks. Finally, in my early twenties, I realized that it didn't matter if other people interpreted me in a way that wasn't true. What mattered was what I knew to be true. With relief, I wrote of this realization:

> For years, I never accurately perceived myself because I was wait-ing for it to come from someone else. I was waiting to always be a Latina or always a gringa, to always be pretty or always be plain, to be exotic or ignored, to be exciting or unappealing. I wanted a con-stant but never found it. The reactions to my looks, my reality, were always extreme. I was waiting for external consistency to garner my own confidence. Ultimately, I realized that the only consistent view that I would get would be my own. My glance in the mirror would have to be accurate. I would have to respect my own assessment. My self-confidence would teach others how to interpret me so I did not have to make a sacrifice. The most important issue was not how other people defined what they saw, but how I defined what I felt, the way I melded my parts, and thus, how I let my Latina and gringa each have her own voice.

So much of our dissatisfaction about our bodies, I believe, stems from our assumption that we *are* our bodies. But we are not our bodies. Our bodies are simply vehicles that take us through this life, that allow us to experience this world, and each was chosen, through genetics, for our par-ticular journey. Our bodies are not who we are. We all know that what we are is a compilation of our heart, our soul, and our mind. Our bodies carry our truth around, they are the lenses through which we experience the world, but they are not us. Our true selves are *rooted within* our bodies.

Today ⟞ Embrace the notion that you are not your body. Accept that your value is greater than your body. If you are at war with your body because you believe it should be something dramatically different, life will be long and unfulfilling. This is not to say you shouldn't care for your body and keep it in good operating order. In fact, you have a responsibility to do that. But if your project in life is to alter your body, you are missing the point. As Erin, one of the students in my body image seminar, recently shared when she had an "Aha!" moment, "Your body is like your vehicle. And if your car's not broken, you don't take it to the shop to fix it just because. You only take it in if it really needs to be fixed. And to carry the analogy further, we all have different needs, which means we all drive different types of vehicles. There's not just one car out there."

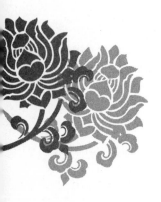

—➤ 12 ◄—

Realize That Your Dissatisfaction Is Not About Your Body

So, if we are not our bodies, then what in the world are we so dissatisfied with? That's just it. Feelings of body hatred, dissatisfaction, and preoccupation are not just about our bodies. It is one thing to wish that we had it in our genes to be a smidge taller. It's another thing to be so consumed by our lack of height that we live our lives differently. In fact, if we find ourselves consumed with body hatred, dissatisfaction, and preoccupation, our issue is likely not about our bodies at all. It's about something else that has kept us from maintaining perspective about our perceived imperfections.

Today —➤ In your *Beautiful You* journal, consider that your dissatisfaction is not about your body. When you accept that thought, what comes to mind? What is your dissatisfaction really about? What is it trying to tell you? What part of your life could you address to foster more overall contentment?

— 13 —

Define Beautiful

When I was doing research for *Hijas Americanas*, I asked every person I interviewed to define beautiful. Their answers never relied on physical appearance. Instead, they talked about confidence, compassion, and self-awareness. Several questions later, I asked each person if she considered herself beautiful. "Absolutely not," they always answered. At this point, I had been talking to each woman about fairly personal information for more than an hour. I didn't know her, necessarily, but I had been honored with intimate details about her life and her sense of self, and I could absolutely discern whether she matched her own definition of beautiful. And when she did, I would call her on it. Always gently, I would say I found it interesting that she defined beauty in this particular way and that, over the course of the interview, I had seen those traits exhibited by her in these distinct ways. And yet, I'd continue, I was struck that while she was willing to label other people in her life beautiful, she wasn't willing to judge herself on those same standards and give herself that same grace. Those moments were always my favorite ones in the interviews, and I often had women email me afterwards to comment on and thank me for that specific part of our conversation.

Today —— In your *Beautiful You* journal, write down what the word *beautiful* means to you. When are you compelled to use that word to describe a person? What has informed your definition? Knowing and owning our personal definitions of beauty is an essential step in celebrating one's own brilliance.

DAY

— 14 —

Banish "Have You Lost Weight?" From Your Vocabulary

There's a person I see about every two months who often asks me the same question: "Have you lost weight?" What I have noticed is that the question always comes on the days she sees me in regular-life clothes instead of workout clothes. I look more polished on those days, and looking more polished, it turns out, means looking like I've lost weight. Except I never have lost weight, and it makes the conversation awkward. Hanging in the air is the notion that she thought I *needed* to lose weight and would approve of anything I had lost. So I say no, and she continues to insist that surely I have. If I were more insecure about my weight, I'd carry it with me for awhile. Instead, I just use it as a reminder that the question "Have you lost weight?" creates a lose-lose situation for both parties involved.

Today — Make a commitment to banish "Have you lost weight?" from your vocabulary. Our weight shouldn't be up for grabs in conversation— as either question or commentary. When you ask someone, out of the blue, "Have you lost weight?" you leave her wondering what you think of her and why. It's one thing if your sister reveals to you that she wants to get healthier and hopes that you'll help her on her journey. But it's another thing entirely to ask such a loaded question of someone whose goals, insecurities, needs, and medical issues you know nothing about. If what you are thinking is really "You look great!" then just say that, with no qualifiers attached. By banishing weight-loss comments from your vocabulary, you keep yourself from perpetuating the notion that someone's weight and body size are fair game for discussion and up for both grabs and judgment.

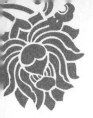

— 15 —

Have a Child Draw a Picture

In January 2009, we adopted a baby boy from Ethiopia. When we traveled to Ethiopia for the adoption, we were fortunate to be in the company of three other wonderful families who used the same agency to facilitate their adoptions. The Andersons were one of those families. Jillian and Ashley adopted two older boys, Morgan and Parker, who were around seven and ten, respectively.

As the months passed post-adoption, we shared stories, asked each other questions, offered listening ears. We met up when we were traveling, followed each other's blogs, sent photos.

Morgan and Parker had experienced a great deal in their young lives, but Jillian and Ashley were absolutely committed to seeing them through the transition process so that they could become their true and best selves, grow in the love offered to them, and relish in the possibility available to them.

The first month home, Jillian had the boys look in the mirror and draw portraits of themselves. Nine months later, they repeated the exercise. The original portraits lacked vitality: the boys were standing still in them, their clothing nondescript, their mouths drawn as straight lines. The later drawings were a revelation: a mouth curled into a smile here, a smiley-face t-shirt there, a running body, a moving mouth, Morgan as Spiderman, Parker as Captain America. The boys in these pictures jumped off the page, filled with energy, aliveness, and spirit. There was a sense of knowing there, a self-knowledge that had been awakened under Jillian and Ashley's gentle and constant care.

Today —— Have a child in your life draw a self-portrait. Give him or her a mirror if that will help. Then hold onto that picture. In the coming months, be as deliberate about guiding that child's journey as you are about yours, then marvel at the difference between today's picture and a later one.

— 16 —

Draw a Picture of Yourself

Jillian's exercise for Morgan and Parker isn't just for kids. It can be revealing for adults as well.

Today —— In your *Beautiful You* journal, draw a picture of yourself as you perceive yourself today. Be as honest as possible in your rendering so you have a true gauge of your self-image for later reflection.

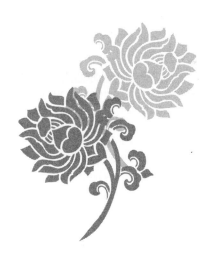

— 17 —

Replace What You Heard

We often fear bringing past hurts to the surface of consciousness because we are scared of the damage they could do—yet subconsciously we have been processing those hurts all along. Many people with self-esteem or body issues will reveal that those issues began because of something they heard from someone else. A coach, a brother, a critical friend, or maybe their mom repeated something negative often enough that they started to listen to the racket. The truth is that we internalize what we hear. If we hear negative, we internalize negative.

Dr. Amy Combs is a clinical psychologist and the director of the Charlotte Center for Balanced Living, a holistic treatment center in Charlotte, North Carolina, that specializes in disordered eating. Dr. Combs encourages her clients to begin processing and reconciling past experiences, so they can move past them, using the exercise below.

Today —— Consider the negative messages about yourself that are in your head and ask yourself, "Is this my voice or someone else's?"

Says Combs, "A lot of people feel good about everything in their lives except their body. One of the first things we can do is to ask these questions of ourselves: Whose voice is it? Where did it come from? Why does it make sense for me to talk to myself like that?"

Next, Combs offers questions like these. "If this negative message was shared with you at a younger age, how would you re-parent yourself? What do you think your friend was missing in her life that made her say that? Do you think this is really what your brother thought, or was it how he thought he could get you the most upset? What was the goal?"

Whatever you may have been told, replace it right now with what you wish you had heard.

— 18 —

Have a Comeback

One of the first topics we tackle in the body image seminar is *Parents, Peers, and Body Image*. And while I inevitably worry that since it's the beginning of the semester, no one will share when it comes time for class discussion, that has never been the case. Unfortunately, our families and friends have had a significant impact on our sense of ourselves. I say "unfortunately" because that impact is often not positive. My students remember their father's jabs, their grandmother's backhanded compliments, and their mother's pressuring. They remember what their friends said to or about them. They anticipate that it will come up again. And so, with every class discussion on *Parents, Peers, and Body Image*, we do the same exercise. After I talk about the importance of teaching people how to treat us, and stress that we can set limits for the people in our lives, we, as a class, brainstorm appropriate comebacks for the negative things that continue to haunt us.

My favorite? A young woman described how her mother told her she would be so much happier if she just lost twenty pounds. The comeback someone came up with in class: "Don't you mean that you would be so much happier, Mom, if I just lost twenty pounds?"

Today —— Think of the jabs you sometimes hear from friends and family members. Perhaps they are about your appearance, your relationship status, or whether or not you have kids. Now take some time to come up with the perfect comeback. What can you say, the next time it happens, to let that critical person know that you would like to be treated differently or that your body is off limits for discussion? Worried that you'll forget the comeback? Write it down in your *Beautiful You* journal. Periodically practice the comeback, in your mind and out loud, so that you are ready when you need to use it.

— 19 —

Nourish Your Body

I fell incredibly ill in my mid-twenties. Wiped out, I saw my doctor repeatedly as I tried to find an explanation for the fainting episodes, forgetfulness, nausea, shakiness, and fuzzy thinking that plagued me.

"You just turned twenty-five," he told me. I stared at him, dumbfounded that quarter-centuryness was his diagnosis.

Finally, after four months of my badgering, he scheduled a glucose tolerance test. It turned out I was hypoglycemic, meaning that I suffered from chronic low blood sugar.

I made an appointment with a nutritionist and what I learned in the months that I worked with her is this: food is medicine. My poor eating habits had evolved because I was consumed by teaching and coaching and did not have time to put any effort into nourishment. Actually, I didn't have time *not* to nurture my body. I didn't have time for emergency room visits, passing out in public and having to explain myself, memory loss, or the decline in my function. As I munched on grapes with almonds for my midday snack, as I sipped water instead of soda, as I prepared peanut butter and jelly sandwiches on whole wheat, I began to realize how much better I felt when I nourished my body with real nutrients and not overly processed food. Even now, I know when I've been eating too much crap because I immediately start to feel run-down. Food really is medicine, and your body responds with energy and vitality when you treat it well. Feeling good becomes its own reward.

Today —— Nourish your body with healthy foods. Watch your intake of processed foods and sugary drinks, try to eat as "cleanly" as possible (do you recognize all the ingredients on the food label?), and observe how your body feels when you make good food choices. Are you avoiding the late afternoon slump? Do you have more energy throughout the day? Are you happier? Eating in a way that nourishes your body is a great way to boost your sense of well-being. And if you slip up, be kind to yourself and eat well with the next meal. It's okay to take pleasure in indulging on occasion without feeling guilty.

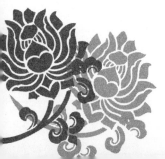

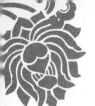

— 20 —

Consider the Time You've Lost

For years, my hair was simply wide. Not curly, certainly, and not stick-straight, just thick and frizzy. Then, the summer between my freshman and sophomore year of high school, I washed my hair one morning and it dried curly. It has been curly ever since. For a while, it was too wild, too big, too out of control, and I didn't know how to work with it. This was before there were all the products for curly hair, so I did the only thing I knew to do: I straightened it. Almost every day, I put an hour or more into drying my hair wide because that is what I knew. Then one day, rushing to dry my hair because I had so many other things I needed to do, it occurred to me that in just one year of drying my hair 300 times, I had lost 300 hours of doing something else—anything else—besides trying to get my hair to behave in a way that was contrary to its will. That struck me as sad and ridiculous and a shame. So I put down the hair dryer and made peace with my hair. Because the truth is, devoting that much time to how I look is contrary to how I want to live.

Today —— Consider the thing that you most obsess over with regard to your appearance, then add up the time you have spent obsessing over it in your life. Now ask yourself the questions I asked myself: Is it worth it? Is your hair, your makeup, your outfit deserving of that much of the time you have left in your life? Can you let a little of it go? Can you start today?

— 21 —

Consider How You Have Been Championed

Just as it is valuable to reflect on what you have learned from past experiences that hurt you, it is also important to reflect on what you have learned from past experiences where you were championed—either by yourself or someone else.

Today —— Answer these questions in your *Beautiful You* journal. Are there moments in your life where you have felt championed? What were those experiences like and what did you learn from them?

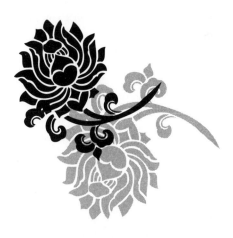

— 22 —

Paint a Plate

When I taught high school, one of my students struggled with particularly difficult lows, and we often talked during these times. During one conversation, I asked her what could still bring a smile to her face. As soon as I asked the question, her face brightened with recognition. She told me how her boyfriend's mother had a plate that said "You are Special" on it, and when anyone in the family, my student included, did something special—earned their driver's license, made an A on a test, scored in an athletic match or kept someone else from scoring—the plate came out for that person to use at the next meal. My student, who was outstanding but, like many young women today, struggled with knowing her worth, loved the times when the plate made its way in front of her. In those moments, she felt seen, appreciated, beautiful, and, indeed, special.

Today — Stop by a pottery-painting store and paint a "You are Special" plate. Once it has been glazed, use it to celebrate the brilliant, beautiful moments in your life and the lives of those you love.

— 23 —

Realize That You Are What You Pay Attention To

Consider this very simple truth. What we pay attention to, what we put energy into, is a statement about what is important to us. It is a reflection of who we are.

Today — In your *Beautiful You* journal, reflect on what you pay attention to, what you give priority, and what you put your energy into on any given day. If we are what we pay attention to, are you comfortable with this reflection of you? If not, how can you adjust your energies to more accurately reflect who you are at your core?

— 24 —

Describe Yourself

Asking my students to describe themselves in their body image autobiographies has also proven to be a very revealing exercise. I am giving them an opportunity to focus on what they feel is important about who they are and their place in the world. Often, they are pleasantly surprised by the answers they discover when they go beyond a superficial physical description.

Today — In your *Beautiful You* journal, describe yourself as completely as you can.

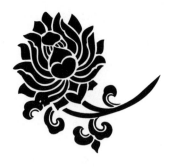

— 25 —

Engage the World

We too often invest in self-loathing—because of everything from our weight to our hair, from our body shape to our skin color. The energy we put into all this hating, tweaking, complaining, and trying to erase takes our energy away from engaging in our world. Luminous, shiny hair doesn't make you a better mother. A tan does not make you a better teacher. These things don't change the world. It's what you have inside you—in your soul—that has the makings of an everyday miracle. I find that my sense of self has always come from believing more in what I do than in what I am. Having positive self-esteem is in part about doing things that are worthy of esteem—engaging in acts that build esteem because they are admirable.

Today —— Want to feel better about yourself? Consider this. Investing your time in completing esteemable acts can do much more for your self-esteem than trying the latest mascara or buying skinny jeans. Why measure your worth by a beauty standard that exists on a slippery slope? Over the coming months, we'll talk about specific actions that can help you engage the world in a deliberate way, making both you and the world around you feel better. In your *Beautiful You* journal, reflect on the admirable acts you already do in your life.

— 26 —

End the Rivalry

Sometimes, we are so insecure that we create rivalries that exist only in our minds. We survey the room at a party, passing judgment on who is prettier or skinnier than we are. It is as if the world is one big contest, and we are always a contestant. Television shows like *The Bachelor* just fuel this tendency. In that series, 20 women line up to compete for one bachelor's affection while their rivalry becomes our entertainment. Rivalries unhealthily fuel the mindset that we are "less than" or "more than" other people, when that is not true at all. When we make things into a competition, we create a situation where there are always winners and losers—which means our self-worth swings like a pendulum between anxiety and judgment. The truth, quite simply, is that we are who we are. Other people are simply who they are. There is no competition, no race. There is simply being.

Today — See the women around you as potential allies; let go of *me vs. them* thinking. There isn't just one kind of beauty; there isn't just one perfect body; there isn't just one way to be in the world. The next time you size up another woman, tell yourself, "Let it go." Instead of comparing yourself to her, choose to learn something about her interests and passions. By being less competitive, you will release yourself from the need to feel inadequate or anxious.

Quiet Your Critic

The other day in class, one of my students admitted that though she feels pretty good about herself, she can't stop the commentary in her head about other people—even people she doesn't know, like those she passes in the mall.

Here's the thing. If you have a running commentary going on about other people in your life, it's highly likely that you don't really feel all that good about yourself, deep down inside.

Today —— Pay attention to the commentary in your head and what it says about others. That racket roots you in negativity because it keeps you from seeing the grace in people. It makes you suspicious of others and self-conscious about yourself. *(If I am criticizing everyone I see as I walk through the mall, surely everyone is doing the same thing to me. I wonder what they find wrong with me?)* When you notice yourself being negative about someone else, change your thinking immediately by affirming something about the person instead. Resist the urge to put the person in a box based on your own understanding. Teach yourself to see the goodness in people.

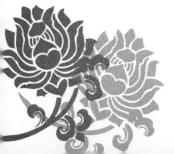

— 28 —

Stop Comparing

Though you are working on ending the rivalry you feel with other women, you might still be inclined to compare yourself to other women, to see where you rank. Let's be honest. What purpose do the comparisons serve? If your barometer for greatness is based on comparing yourself to other women, you are setting yourself up to be unhappy. Why? Because none of those women are you. None of them have your genetics. None of them have your life experiences. None of them face life in the same exact way that you do. And let's face it, the picture-perfect life you see on the outside is not reality anyway.

Today — Turn off the desire to compare. When it happens today, notice it. In your *Beautiful You* journal, reflect on these questions. Who are you comparing yourself to and in what way? What effect is that comparison having on you? What purpose does the comparison serve? Give yourself honest feedback about why you are doing it and then move on. Each time you find yourself in the comparison game, stop and walk yourself through these steps. By gaining an understanding of when and why you make these comparisons, you can begin to gain the upper hand and stop the habit.

— 29 —

Speak Positively

One way that women choose to get power, if they feel like they don't have access to it in other ways, is through gossip. Power can be intoxicating, an addiction in its own right. But what really happens when we gossip is that we poison ourselves. While we think we are boosting our own understanding of ourselves, what we are actually doing is creating our own doubts and insecurities. If we are creating an environment where someone else is unsafe, we subconsciously know that we are condoning the actions of others who speak negatively about us.

Today —— Choose to speak positively about other people and their gifts. Celebrate what they have to offer. By creating a world where all people are embraced and celebrated when people talk about them, you create a more magnanimous place and improve your own sense of self.

— 30 —

Name the Beautiful

We often use a different standard of beauty for ourselves than we do for others. Today, we will examine what we really find beautiful.

Today — In your *Beautiful You* journal, name the people you know that you find beautiful. What is it that makes them so beautiful to you? Do you use the same standard when judging yourself?

— 31 —

Know Your Rights

On December 10, 1948, the General Assembly of the United Nations (which was formed in 1945 with a mission of stopping wars between countries and providing a platform for dialogue) adopted and proclaimed the Universal Declaration of Human Rights, an aspirational document that highlights how this collection of diverse nations would like to see each one of us treated. The hope was that its broad dissemination would keep the atrocities of World War II from happening again. Each year on December 10, the United Nations leads the world in celebrating Human Rights Day, reminding all of us of our own personal dignity and the justice that should be afforded to every one of us. One of the first things to go when we struggle with a negative body image is our own sense of personal dignity. When we can telescope back and see ourselves in a grander sense, a global sense, we can glimpse that dignity and all that it encompasses once again.

Today —— Visit www.un.org/Overview/rights.html and read the Universal Declaration of Human Rights. Make sure that all is quiet around you and that you can fully concentrate on the scope of the act and its potential impact on your life and the lives of others. In your *Beautiful You* journal, write down the article that most strikes you and describe why it stood out. Then relish your rights while considering how you might help these words become a reality for more people around the world by becoming an advocate for the rights of others.

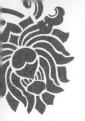

— 32 —

Celebrate Your Birth Day

Do a set of regular push-ups.
Take my parents to visit family in Puerto Rico.
Work with turtles.
Complete a century bicycle ride.
Raise at least $5,000 for cancer research.

Every year, I celebrate my birthday by writing a list. It started as a simple dare. Find something to do outside of your job, I told myself in that third year of teaching, when my work hours stretched from six in the morning until ten at night, or you will end up celebrating your sixtieth birthday wondering where your life went.

My first list was written in the days leading up to my twenty-fifth birthday. Scrawled across the pages of a journal, I listed the twenty-five things I wanted to do before I turned twenty-six. Back then, it was mostly a practical venture. I started to run, paid off student loans, saved money, took a CPR class. Each year, the list grew a little more adventurous, balancing the trivial with the important, the safe with the stretches. I learned to paint, went kayaking, sang karaoke. I took other risks, like submitting my poetry and nonfiction essays to literary magazines and performing in *The Vagina Monologues*. Each checkmark on the list made me feel more alive, made me more certain of myself.

I was living more fully, with both practical challenges and extraordinary experiences informing my growth. Learning to swim made me safer. Learning CPR helped me keep others safe. Scaling a 5.7c peak in rock climbing made me reach deep inside to find reservoirs of strength and endurance. Today, I am more athletic. I have helped my family, traveled and experienced other cultures, made new friends, engaged in my community, developed artistic skills, invested in issues that are dear to me, become better read, become more grounded.

I have never completed all the tasks on any year's list, but the fact that the list exists lures me into looking it over, making plans, and checking things off. I know that I live better and more dramatically because the list exists. At the end of each "birth" year, I evaluate the list. I recall each experience and think about its significance to me. I consider who I have been and who I am becoming, and I decide whether an unmet goal should go on the next year's list or if it is no longer calling to me. The list is a reminder that my life is not the sum total of my appearances. It is the sum total of my experiences. Regardless of what I decide to add to each list, each year is cloaked in adventure, compassion, self-improvement, and satisfaction. My list is a gift to myself, a celebration of life, something that keeps me living out loud.

Today ⊶ In your *Beautiful You* journal, begin to draft your own birthday to-do list. How close is your birthday to today? If it's at least six months away, write a list of things to do that adds up to half your age. Less than six months? Write a list that represents a quarter or third of your age. Now take just one item from that list and figure out when and how you are going to accomplish it.

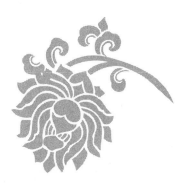

— 33 —

Complete These Sentences

Reflection helps you grow; it nudges you a step closer to your best self as you reflect on and interpret what has passed before you. Journaling allows you to see the familiar in new ways, and it doesn't require a significant time commitment to be productive and rewarding.

Today —— Finish these five sentences in your *Beautiful You* journal.

Someone who energizes me is . . .

I am taking a greater interest in . . .

I am yearning for . . .

I am proud of . . .

I believe in . . .

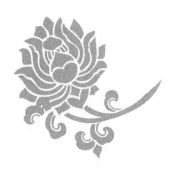

— 34 —

Use Twenty-Five Words

Seeing ourselves in a way that is not just linked to our physical appearance or the roles we play in our lives is essential. After all, we are much more than the way we look or the way we interact with or provide for other people. By better understanding our totality, we can more fully embrace our entire selves.

Today —— In your *Beautiful You* journal, describe yourself, in twenty-five words or less, without using any physical descriptors or naming any of your roles. Don't overthink it. Just write your sentence in a minute or less. When you read what you've written, you might discover a simple truth about yourself—a mission, a vision, or a crucible.

Need an example? Here are two such descriptors I have written about myself:

I am a woman who is proud of her history, aspires to use her creativity positively, and looks forward to her future.

I am a woman who is suddenly aware that I can control my destiny by creating the day that I most wish to have.

— 35 —

Watch the Dove Videos

Dove began its Campaign for Real Beauty and Self-Esteem Fund after their study, "The Real Truth about Beauty," revealed that only 2 percent of women around the world described themselves as beautiful. One aspect of the campaign has been the provocative, thoughtful videos that Dove produced in an effort to get women to think differently about beauty.

Today —— Visit www.dove.us; choose *Features* and *Videos* and watch "Onslaught," "Evolution," and "Amy" to gain some perspective on beauty standards and the beauty industry.

DAY

— 36 —

Don't Make Unrealistic Comparisons

When I was writing *Hijas Americanas*, I met a young woman who spent more than $100 each month buying fashion magazines and then pouring over the pages of each issue, searching for someone who looked like her. If she could find someone, she imagined that she would cut herself a little slack on her journey to physical perfection. But she never did, so she put herself through the awful throes of bulimia instead, purging through exercise and vomiting.

What struck me as she told this story was that she was comparing herself to images that were not even real. Most of the bodies we see represented in magazines are achieved through artificial means. I've heard many a professional actress or model say that it takes hours to make them look like the public idea of themselves, and that is valuable information for all of us to have. In the best-case scenario, a celebrity looks like that after hours spent with professional makeup artists and hair stylists, under perfectly arranged lighting, and with Photoshop and airbrush enhancements. In the worst-case scenario, a celebrity looks like that after all of the above and significant cosmetic surgery.

Today —— Learn about Photoshopping so that you'll stop comparing yourself to media images. Enter "Photoshop before and after" in a search engine to learn more about the alterations that take place through computer manipulation. Understand that the photos you see in a magazine are actually stylized images—ideas we are being presented after much work on and off the set to make them look that way—not like the actual photos we get out of our camera.

DAY

— 37 —

Get Fitted

You've seen it on *Oprah* and read it in your magazines. Most women are wearing the wrong bra size. And the wrong bra impacts both how you feel (underwires that dig into your sides are enough to make any woman crazy) and how your clothes look, which impacts your sense of confidence.

Today —— Stop by a department store with a reputable lingerie department or a specialty lingerie store. Get fitted for a bra to make sure you are wearing the right size. If you aren't, try on a few different styles in your correct size. See which one you like best for its look and feel, and invest in yourself by buying one.

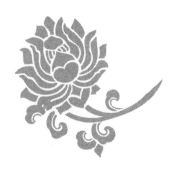

— 38 —

Identify Your Go-To Girl

Every woman should have a person she goes to when she needs understanding, perspective, comfort, or commiseration. It's the friend you can call to say, "I just need to bitch about something" or "I can't believe this happened" or anything else in between. Sharing your problems with that one go-to person helps you put your worries in perspective, offers you fresh solutions, and can help halt the cycle of negative thoughts.

I've learned that if I call a friend (or my sister) early in any cycle of worry or stress, my anxiety dissipates much faster. It loses the strength it has over me, which boosts my resolve and sense of self. It allows me to move forward more quickly and to feel more empowered. This person doesn't just need to be around to hear your grievances. She can also be your partner on your journey to self-satisfaction, someone you can check in with as you encounter growth opportunities and consider new possibilities.

Today — Identify your Go-To Girl. Who is that one person you can turn to when life hands you a curveball or when you are considering a significant next step? Who will treat anything you tell her with confidentiality while giving you good advice, insight, and perspective? Who would be able to help you gather your thoughts? If you want, call the friend you are thinking of. Tell her you are looking for someone with whom you can share your concerns and possibilities, and that you'd like it to be her. Ask if this would be okay with her. Let her know she can count on you for the same support. Then next time life throws you for a loop and you feel your stomach knotting up, call your Go-To Girl and feel the anxiety dissipate as you talk to her.

— 39 —

Have Someone Else Make a Resolution For You

I don't typically make resolutions, but as January 2009 was nearing, I started thinking about them in a way that I don't usually. And while there were plenty of things for me to gain resolve about, none of them were that interesting to me. I keep my bad habits because I like them just fine, thank you.

So I decided to ask my husband to set a New Year's resolution for me. I felt sure he would focus on one of the bad habits I really do like, but he didn't. Instead, he wanted me to resolve to wash my breakfast dish as soon as I was done with it, or put it in the dishwasher, rather than leave it in the sink until it was time to deal with my lunch dish, too. (Can you tell we were both working in home offices?) It was an easy thing to do, and it was actually refreshing and affirming that out of all the things that he could have asked, he chose something so simple.

Oftentimes we are our own biggest critics, and our inner dialogue about what we should and could do is paralyzing, moving us further away from our own brilliance. If only we could see our behaviors through someone else's lens. Sometimes it is best to let someone else see you with their smallest eye and guide you in taking a step that moves you forward with grace.

Today — Ask a loved one to suggest a simple resolution for you to tackle in the coming weeks. Now make room in your heart and attempt it.

DAY

— 40 —

Go to Bed Earlier

For the first several months after we became new parents, our baby boy awoke fifteen to twenty times a night. Soon, I had lost luster in both my personality and skin tone. I was exhausted, I looked it, and the beating I was taking from lack of sleep affected everything in my life. Then, one night, our baby woke just three times. I was amazed at how significantly different I felt after just one night of better sleep—I was surprised that it could make that much of a difference that fast. After a few more three-wake-up nights, I was convinced that sleep was one of the essential steps in feeling my best, so I started thinking about how I could get more. While I knew that going to bed earlier was the answer, I was reluctant to give up that time I used for late night tinkering. Ultimately, though, I realized that I got far more out of sleeping than I did from squeezing out work with a waning spirit after putting the baby down for the night.

Today ⟶ Go to bed earlier! Figure out what time you need to lie down to get eight hours of sleep—meaning you should probably go lights-out with more than eight-and-a-half hours between you and that morning alarm, to account for the time you might spend lying awake and stressing. Keep that commitment to yourself tonight.

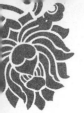

— 41 —

Accept Your Imperfections

Not one of us is perfect, and yet we often worry that if we don't keep the illusion of our own perfection going, someone might discover our horrifying secret—that everything we do isn't brilliant. Never have my imperfections been more pronounced than in the months following the arrival of our baby boy. Sleep deprived and distracted, I forgot birthdays, was slower to return phone calls, and just generally fell behind. There was no hiding it. Ultimately, I gave up trying to figure out how I could have missed a detail here and there and just accepted that I did. Forgiving myself and recognizing that no one expected me to be perfect allowed me to experience much more joy during that time. The truth is that people aren't fired or unfriended or dismissed for being imperfect. If you are unlikable, that's another story. But imperfection is just refreshing and way relatable.

Today —— Give up the perfection facade and just be who you are. If you read an email wrong, laugh about it. If you missed a detail, apologize. If you don't understand, ask a follow-up question. By allowing yourself to be who you are in any moment, you begin to recognize that you are just enough. And by embracing who you are—strengths and challenges entwined—you begin to celebrate the beauty within you.

DAY

— 42 —

Finish These Sentences

Sometimes, we just need to remind ourselves of what's possible; we just need to relish in the new beginnings that we can create.

Today ⟶ In your *Beautiful You* journal, finish these sentences.

I can . . .

I will . . .

I expect . . .

I look forward to . . .

I hope . . .

I wish . . .

I plan . . .

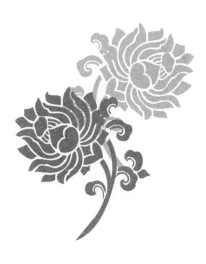

DAY

— 43 —

Get Political

There is a sociopolitical lesson in the consideration of beauty standards and body image. When we become consumed with our appearance, we are left with little room to think about much else. And when we are unable to become fully possessed of ourselves, when we are unable to recognize what makes us great or unique and instead wallow in what makes us—in our minds—"less than" or "different," we are, in truth, oppressed.

Beauty standards are, in many ways, a political issue. As long as you can be kept obsessed, you can be kept oppressed.

Today —— Recognize that by being consumed by your appearance and the ways you do not measure up to someone else's beauty standard, you are holding yourself back from being consumed by the calling of your life, from embracing your great gladness and giving it to the world. Imagine your life without the beauty obsession. Would you have time and energy for something else? If so, begin exploring that something else now.

— 44 —

Embrace Your Passion

Recently, I gave a talk to the health department employees in my community who work with teenage mothers and mothers-to-be.

One of them asked, "What can we do to help these girls continue on the path to high school graduation and what might come after?"

"We need to empower these girls to find their passions," I answered.

One of the greatest gifts we can give ourselves is a *passion*, something that brings us so much joy and satisfaction that we can't help but feel successful when we are doing it. When we are doing something we are passionate about, we can't help but feel like we have something to offer.

Becoming passionate about something, and then investing time and energy in it, adds vitality to our lives. Vitality builds self-esteem and confidence. But embracing a passion also does something else. It motivates us to take time for ourselves. And when we make the things we are passionate about a priority—especially if our passions positively impact someone else—we make ourselves better.

Today ——— Consider what you love to do. Are you happiest when gardening? Do you love working with dogs? Does cooking bring you comfort and contentment? Whatever it is that fires you up, make room in your life—not just to accommodate it, but to embrace it. Don't excuse away your need to engage in it. Instead, think of it as a vital part of who you are and realize that by engaging in your passion, you give the world both your gift and the joy of watching you become energized. Not sure what your passion is? Ask your friends what they love, what fires them up. If something sounds particularly interesting, ask if you can tag along the next time they are embracing their passion. Maybe it will speak to you too.

— 45 —

Own Your Body

Molly Barker, founder of Girls on the Run International, is a woman I greatly admire. Through Girls on the Run programs, girls from third grade through middle school learn to honor themselves, embrace the concept of team, and become empowered to change their worlds. They are taught to understand that they are not objects and that the ownership of their bodies is theirs alone.

When Molly talks about her inspiration for Girls on the Run, she is honest about her own struggles. She also gives a name to a phenomenon that perhaps we have noticed but never classified. The "Girl Box" is the place that girls put themselves—and society puts girls—as they come of age. Inside that box, girls find that they are inclined to morph into who they think they should be, rather than who they naturally are. In the Girl Box, body objectification begins in earnest. Society begins to judge girls on a universal standard, and girls begin to realize that by objectifying their own bodies, they can gain power or access.

Today ——— Own your body. Wrap your mind around the concept that you are the one who can choose to either *use* your body or *own* your body. Understand that your body can be a tool that enables you to help yourself and other people—that it can expand your universe, that it does not have to fit into a box of someone else's construct. Act today from a place that shows that you own your body. By operating in a way that shows the choices you make about your body (what you wear, what you eat, how you carry yourself, the way you care for yourself) are yours alone, you take ownership of what is rightfully yours.

— 46 —

Do Something You Enjoy

When I teach my journaling workshops, I ask participants to make a list of the things they enjoy doing. Then, next to each item, I ask them to write the date on which they last pursued that activity. Taking pleasure in life, after all, reduces our stress, increases our endorphins, and gives us an overall sense of well-being.

Today —— In your *Beautiful You* journal, take five minutes to list everything that you enjoy doing, along with the date that you last did each thing. If you can't remember the exact date, an approximate one is fine (for example, "horseback riding, when I was fourteen" or "surfing, the summer of 2005"). Now look over your list and consider why you have denied yourself some of these pleasures for so long. Choose one thing you can do today.

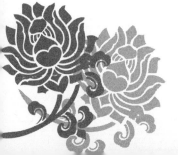

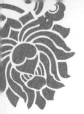

— 47 —

Admire Yourself Doing Something You Love

Sometimes a simple, physical memento goes a long way in reminding us of the pleasure of living and the joy our bodies bring us.

Today — Find a photograph that shows you doing something you love. It doesn't have to be recent, but it should be a photograph that brings a smile to your face when you see it. Display the photo in an area where you spend a significant amount of time: on the bulletin board above your desk, in a picture frame on your kitchen windowsill, in a frame on your bathroom counter. Each time your eyes travel to that photograph, smile in recognition of the joy your body has brought you.

— 48 —

Get a Real Sense of Your Body

A close friend was recently treated for eating disorders. As part of her treatment, her therapist asked her to speak directly to a handful of different friends about her condition. My friend showed each of us a chart that included silhouettes of women in a variety of shapes, from one that appeared fairly underweight to one that looked fairly overweight. She asked us which silhouette we thought came closest to representing her own, then she shared with us which frame she had chosen for herself and why. What she learned over the course of this exercise was that her loved ones shared a similar impression of her body—one that was very different than her own. This exercise helped her to see that her perception of her body might not be grounded in reality, and it allowed her to become kinder to herself as she continued her treatment.

Today — Depending on your height, get two or three pieces of poster board (or a long piece of butcher paper). Tape the boards together, then draw your impression of your body on them. Next, have someone trace the outline of your body on the same boards. Compare the two silhouettes. Now reflect on the following questions in your *Beautiful You* journal. Are the two silhouettes similar in size? Do you have a realistic sense of your body size? Or was it skewed one way or the other? What surprises you from this exercise? What has this exercise taught you?

DAY

— **49** —

Consider Your Personal Locus of Control

The concept of "locus of control" was developed by psychologist Julian Rotter in the 1950s. Locus of control refers to an individual's perception of how much control she has over her destiny. Are the outcomes of our lives and actions based on what we do, or are they based on some external factors we have no control over?

"A realized personal locus of control is empowering," explains Dr. Amy Combs, a clinical psychologist and director of the Charlotte Center for Balanced Living. "It encourages; it mandates us to use our voice and be seen and heard in the world. It gives us a sense of agency and purpose. It also allows us to take personal responsibility for our successes instead of assuming 'it just happened' or 'it was luck.' It encourages us to plot the course of our lives with both short-term and long-term aspirations and goals."

Having an *external* locus of control means you believe that your behavior is guided by external circumstances; having an *internal* locus of control means you believe your behavior is guided by your personal decisions and effort. When an internal locus of control is matched with a person's competence and a realistic sense of influence, good things can happen.

Today —— In your *Beautiful You* journal, consider your personal locus of control. Who or what is controlling your destiny—and why?

Dr. Combs suggests that you ask yourself a question like this, filling in the blank with some action: What might happen if I . . . ?

"Then," she says, "do it. Many times this may involve a risk of some sort. An internal locus of control encourages us to put ourselves out there and take advantage of opportunities."

Wherever you are right now, it is possible to develop a stronger internal locus of control, along with the skills that complement it. By asking yourself what would happen if you went forward with exerting your desire and authority when you are tempted to let external factors control the situation, you build your ability to act from your own sense of self and confidence. Over the course of this year, you will be lead through many tasks and questions that will help you reach a satisfying personal locus of control.

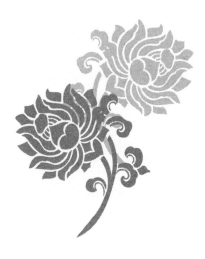

— 50 —

Ask Others to Define Beauty

We don't really talk about beauty with those whom we are close to. But those conversations can often be quite illuminating, allowing us to put body image in perspective by reflecting on the opinions of people that we trust.

Today —— Ask five people you are close to how they would define beauty. After you've heard all five definitions, consider what they have in common and ways in which they differ. Now write your own definition in your *Beautiful You* journal. By seeing the way five people you love look at beauty, you see that the concept has both profoundly individualistic and universal characteristics.

— 51 —

Remind Yourself How Subjective Beauty Is

When *Thelma and Louise* came out, my sister developed a crush on Brad Pitt.

Seriously? I thought. He just looks dirty to me.

To this day, Brad Pitt has never done it for me. While my post-college roommate always loved Tom Cruise, I didn't even bother to watch *Top Gun*. But if Matthew Fox or George Clooney walked into the room, I wouldn't be able to find words.

We all know there isn't one right way to look, just as there is no one path to beauty. What appeals to any one of us—physically and emotionally—is incredibly subjective. But sometimes we need something to very deliberately remind us of that truth.

Today — Engage your friends or loved ones in a conversation about some of your favorite things. What are your favorite movies, books, television shows? Who are your favorite female and male actors? Listen to people's answers and their reasoning, and don't try to change their opinions. Instead, relish the recognition that people don't perceive things in the same ways. By embracing the idea that beauty is inherently subjective—that it is impossible to please all people with just one aesthetic or sensibility— you can more easily accept and embrace the value of your own uniqueness.

DAY

—• 52 •—

People Watch

Walking through an airport always reminds me how important it is to walk through life with our eyes wide open. Settled into where we live or work or exercise, we begin to believe that people look, dress, and act in just a few ways—the ways that are the cultural norms wherever we are. Landing in an airport, especially an international airport, cracks everything back open for us, reigniting our appreciation for the diversity of looks and styles that exist.

Today —• Go somewhere like a crowded public park, an amusement park, or a shopping mall and just people watch. Remember to turn off the judge and critic in your head—the one that would compare your hair, your weight, your style to the person walking by you or the one that would be cynical about someone else's appearance—and just watch. Take in the great diversity that exists and allow it to broaden your understanding of beauty.

Look 'Em in the Eyes

So much of our confidence is projected through our eyes. Avoiding eye contact is just one way of communicating to the world that you want to be invisible. It also communicates to the person whose eyes you are avoiding that he or she isn't worthy of being seen, even if you don't mean to send that message.

Today —— Slow down and look into the eyes of every person you speak to—at the coffee shop, the deli, the newspaper stand, the gas station; in your office, at home, wherever you go. Test yourself. After every single interpersonal exchange, ask yourself what color the other person's eyes were—and make sure you can answer.

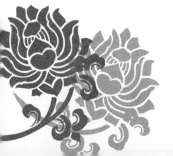

— 54 —

Reflect on Your Self-Care

Self-care is an important part of loving our bodies. In their body image autobiographies, I ask my students to share how they care for themselves each day and how they show their bodies disrespect each day. They talk about their eating habits, patterns of smoking or excessive drinking or lack of sleep and whether or not they exercise. The exercise illuminates the imbalance between self-caring and self-harming behaviors, and it usually sparks a positive change.

Today —— In your *Beautiful You* journal, reflect on the ways you care for yourself each day. Now think about the ways that you show yourself a lack of care each day. Finally, name five tangible things you can start doing each day to care for yourself. What preparations are needed, and when can you start doing these things? Begin as soon as you can.

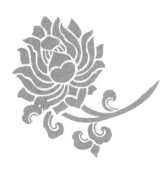

— 55 —

Diversify Your Interests

Ⅰf your entire sense of self comes from the way you look, then it's safe to say you will feel defeated on days when your hair isn't looking its best, your outfit doesn't fit quite right, or your skin has a breakout. It's like the saying that you shouldn't put all your eggs in one basket—you certainly don't want your self-esteem to come from just one place. Having multiple sources of self-worth—a job you enjoy, friends and family you love, a cause that makes you feel passionate, a hobby that absorbs you, a community that you invest in—will ultimately lead to a happier, healthier, more confident you.

Today — Consider the sources of your self-esteem. In your *Beautiful You* journal, explore these questions. Does your sense of worth come from multiple places? If not, in what ways can you diversify your life portfolio to live in a way that affirms you and your gifts daily?

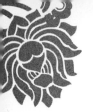

Volunteer

When I went to college, I realized pretty quickly that I was different from many of my peers. Perhaps I could have stayed in that place where I was always aware that my body and hair and even socioeconomic class were different. But I didn't because I had a scholarship that required me to volunteer at least ten hours a week—and volunteering, it turned out, was what brought out the best in me.

While I could have been losing confidence over my perceived differences, I was instead gaining confidence over my demonstrated strengths. And while my experience being engaged in the community taught me many global lessons, it also taught me this very personal one: self-confidence flourishes when you are not focusing on yourself. When you spend too much time obsessing over your weight or nose or curls or skin color, you lose the ability to really engage in the lives and happenings around you because all you are thinking about and worrying about is you. Shifting attention from your own worries and concerns to someone else's can give you perspective and an education about the world, and it might very well lead you to your passion (as it did for me). Dwelling on our perceived shortcomings only leads to personal unhappiness. Looking outward instead is a gift to both ourselves and our world.

Today —— Arrange a date to volunteer. You may know exactly where you'd like to volunteer, but if you don't, visit www.volunteermatch.org or www.idealist.org, or call your local United Way for ideas. If you are already volunteering, consider whether or not the experience has been fulfilling. If not, reassess. If so, consider adding a few more responsibilities or hours.

DAY

— 57 —

Schedule Breaks

I remember once being so busy in high school that I would go to bed at night, exhausted, and think, "Maybe something mildly bad will happen, like a really bad flu or a minor car accident, so that I can take a little bit of time off." It is so sad for me to look back and see how powerless I felt about getting off the merry-go-round of life periodically in order to regroup and reenergize. When I went off to college, I deliberately thought, *I am not signing up for much my first semester,* and I knew I was trying to recover from the burnout that's inevitable when you go, go, go. Unfortunately, I didn't learn my lesson at eighteen, and I've let myself burn out a few times since then. What I have found to be the best medicine is exactly what I wanted a bout of flu to give me back in high school: permission to take a break. The reality is that we control our destiny, our happiness, our pace, and the way we perceive our world. We have the right to change our pace, and, in order to have the stamina for what we already must do, we sometimes must also rest.

Today — Look at your calendar right now and schedule a few different types of breaks. First, schedule a one- to two-hour break sometime in the next two weeks. You can go to a movie during that break or get your nails done or nap, whatever strikes you; you just have to be off for that time. Go ahead, block that time off in red in your electronic or paper planner.

Next, schedule a day where nothing will be officially scheduled. You will just wake up and choose what you want to do at any given moment. Finally, schedule a couple days off. The idea here is to give yourself breathing room, to facilitate the quiet and stillness you need to listen, observe, enjoy, and simply be. It is in doing those things that you come fully into yourself.

— 58 —

Accept That There's No Such Thing as a Joke about Someone's Body

When I was teaching high school, I had strict rules about respecting one another in my classroom. My students were never allowed to say "Shut up" because it extinguished someone else's voice. We could laugh together, sure, but it always had to be together and not at one another. One day during my Advanced Placement United States History class, a group of students got up in front of the room to give a presentation. John, a football player and wrestler who was in the group, started to do push-ups against my desk while waiting to present. Without thinking, I said, "Alright, tough guy, we know you're strong. Now, show us what you have in your head." John blushed and quit the push-ups, but one of the other boys in my classroom quickly turned to me. "Moli, that's not like you to embarrass one of us." And it wasn't; he was absolutely right. Right then, I apologized to John, who took it in stride, but that experience made me doubly sure to keep body humor far away from my lips.

Today — Bite your tongue. Take notice when you think about using humor to discuss someone else's body, and don't give in to the desire, even if it seems like a really funny thing to say. Instead, learn from the experience. While the joke might be funny to you, you don't know how the other person will hear it, and you don't want to reinforce your habit of considering other people's bodies up for grabs. By putting the brakes on your own use of body humor, you won't fuel the fire in others—which means they'll be more likely to put the kibosh on their own attempts at body humor.

— 59 —

Pay a Compliment

A Kansas State University study revealed that one earnest compliment goes a long way in improving one's self-esteem, and it doesn't matter what kind of compliment it is. Maybe this is because we so often see ourselves as imperfect, and a compliment reorders our thinking—for at least a moment—so that we can recognize our worth.

Today —— Pay an earnest compliment to at least five people whose paths you cross. Maybe you love your neighbor's scarf, your coworker's smile, your daughter's artwork, your husband's full-hearted laugh. Whatever it is, whoever it is, notice it and let them know. You'll find that they aren't the only ones who will bask in it. By celebrating others, you are celebrating and bringing out the best in yourself.

— 60 —

Evaluate the Shows You Watch

It is so easy to sit in front of the television and zone out. Before you know it, the whole day has flown by. But in reality, while we may use the term "zoning out" for sitting in front of the television, that's not what is happening. In "The Influence of Television Programs on Appearance and Satisfaction: Making and Mitigating Social Comparisons to Friends," a study published in the 2009 edition of the journal *Sex Roles,* Dr. Stephen Want, an assistant professor in the psychology department at Canada's Ryerson University, revealed that women who watch soap operas or television series where there are many thin and attractive female characters actually perceive their own bodies differently afterwards—even if they say they know better than to compare themselves to television shows. Dr. Want wrote, "People have the tendency to make rapid comparisons of themselves to images on television programs even when they don't think they are being affected."

Today —— Evaluate the television shows you watch so that you know that you are choosing your media actively. Are there any shows that might be impacting your self-esteem? Give up that show (or those shows) this week and fill that time up with an activity that is positive for you, such as taking a walk or talking with a friend. After a couple days pass, see if you are feeling a little bit better about yourself. Have you lost anything by not watching? Can you let the show go for good?

— 61 —

Stop Punishing Yourself

Too many women feel like they are unworthy of enjoying themselves. Instead, they wait, giving themselves goals to achieve before they can engage in something pleasurable.

Today — Don't punish yourself. Stop the "I can have/do/be this when I drop five/fifteen/fifty pounds" language. It's not that you shouldn't want to be healthy. It's that your shape or size shouldn't determine your worth, your sense of self, or your right to take pleasure.

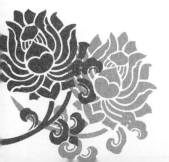

DAY

— 62 —

Treat Yourself

Sometimes when we battle body image and self-esteem issues, we deny ourselves any pleasure, reasoning that when we look the way we want to look or when we accomplish what we think we must accomplish, then we can enjoy ourselves. But radically enforcing deprivation is a form of self-abuse. It is okay to take simple pleasures and to enjoy something in the moment; in fact, that presentness reminds us that life is lived right now and not "one day" in the future. Once we understand that we can fully inhabit and live our lives right now, we come closer to becoming our truest selves.

Today — Treat yourself to a simple, soul-gratifying pleasure. For me, it's a scoop of ice cream or a soak in the tub while reading a good book. For you, it may be something else, something uniquely you. Whatever it is, do something sweet for yourself. Take pleasure in the action and then relish the fact that you can provide yourself with simple happiness.

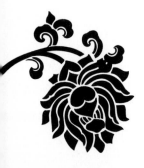

— 63 —

Consider Why the Beauty Industry Exists

For the longest time, I didn't wear makeup. Then in my mid-twenties, I had a makeover with some friends and I was intrigued. I often shopped impulsively, buying things I would never use in my everyday lifestyle. At one point, I owned so much lipstick that I started to use it for artwork. I still own way too much eye shadow, although I have finally admitted to myself that eye shadow is really never going to be my thing. I've probably saved hundreds of dollars in the last few years thanks to that realization.

When I entered "mascara" in an online makeup store's search engine, 211 unique products came up (not counting the color variations available with each product). When there are that many options, how in the world do you decide which one is right for you? Do they do 211 different things to your eyes? The answers to those questions: Who knows and nope.

Personally, I like mascara just fine, but I only own one tube. Because here's the thing about the beauty industry: it exists to make a buck for someone. And making you feel like you have to have the newest mascara product gets you back to the store sooner than if you just waited until your tube of old reliable mascara runs out. The beauty industry relies on our desire for enhancement and breeds on our insecurities. If we can remind ourselves that those ads are about them earning money and not us being imperfect, perhaps we won't buy into it so often.

Today —— Consider what the beauty industry's endgame is: It's their bottom line, not your self-esteem. There's nothing wrong with enjoying makeup. But there is something wrong with relying on makeup to feel good about yourself, and putting all of your hope into products and not your truth. Want to learn even more about the beauty industry? Rent the documentary *Beauty in a Jar*.

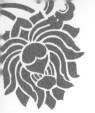

— 64 —

Don't Demonize Food

W hen we demonize food, we also assign it power. A piece of cake becomes a black hole. A pizza slice is the point of no return. A plate of lasagna is the evil stepmother. When we give food that much power, we lose our own power and our perspective. We lose our confidence that we are in control and the faith that we can care for ourselves. By restoring food to its simple role, that of energy provider, we regain our perspective.

Today — Don't demonize food by labeling it bad or evil. Just let it exist as it is and make your choices without those emotional labels attached.

— 65 —

Curtail Negative Behavior

When I was a girl, I hated my nose. And part of hating my nose was spending a fair amount of time looking at it in the mirror, as if I could just will it to change shape. Fortunately for me, life got a lot more interesting and I became a lot less bored. Time with the mirror fell by the wayside when I starting having other things to do. Still, it intrigues me that I obsessed over something I did not have the power to change. It also intrigues me that forgetting about my concern with my nose for a bit—not because anything had changed with it, but because I had other stuff to do—helped me get over it.

Today — Teach yourself to stop body checking. It doesn't serve you, it just keeps you in a heightened state of self-consciousness. Watch for times when you are checking yourself out in mirrors, windows, even shadows. When you catch yourself doing it, take a breath and change your focus. By curtailing the behavior that fuels your obsession, you train yourself to turn off the tape that keeps cycling in your head. Are you having a difficult time curtailing the behavior? Consider talking to someone who specializes in disordered eating behaviors; you might be suffering from body dysmorphic disorder, a condition where an individual focuses a disproportionate amount of time and energy on perceived flaws. With some focused work, you can release yourself from the hold of your obsession.

— 66 —

Sweat It Out

There are different activities that provide me with a sense of well-being, and one of them is working out. Using my body reminds me of what it is really meant to be—a tool to get me through this world. Too often, we view exercise as simply a way to alter the appearance of our bodies, and we don't appreciate the many other ways it is good for us. Exercise is *not* punishment for meals we have had. It is *not* only worth doing if it quickly alters our physique. Exercise is, in fact, a gift of love to our bodies. It improves our sense of well-being and optimizes our heart health. In fact, a study by researchers at the University of Florida found that working out improved body image—even if goals such as weight loss or increased strength were not realized. This may be true because exercise raises our endorphin levels and lowers levels of anxiety and depression, allowing us to look at our bodies in a more positive light.

When I move, I allow my body to do what it does best. Working out rewards me with significant health benefits. It's like good medicine without the aftertaste.

Today —— Instead of working out to change the way your body looks, choose a way to be active that brings you both joy while you are doing it and health benefits when you are done. Take an exercise class, such as indoor cycling or aerobics, or go out for a bike ride or jog. While you're at it, pay particular attention to how you feel; notice how you feel when you are done. Enjoy the sense of well-being and satisfaction that comes from movement.

— 67 —

See Your Body as an Instrument

Athletes know this already. Our bodies are instruments that allow us to accomplish much in our days. They weren't created so that we could just sit back and admire their appearance. They are built for movement, for living, for doing, for being.

Today —— See your body as an instrument, not an ornament. When your mind slips into critiquing how your body looks, stop immediately and celebrate everything your body does. By appreciating the uniqueness of our bodies and their ability to move us through experiencing this world, we can shift our thinking.

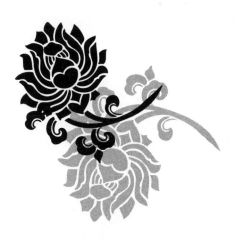

— 68 —

Watch *America the Beautiful*

"Do you feel attractive?"

When Darryl Roberts, a former entertainment reporter in Chicago, approached 200 women on the streets of Chicago and asked them if they felt attractive, only two of them said yes. Yep, just two, meaning 99 percent of the women he approached felt unattractive.

Roberts used the experience to inspire *America the Beautiful,* a documentary that looks at the ways pop culture helps shape our beauty standards and, thus, our insecurities.

Today —— Rent and watch *America the Beautiful.* Then, in your *Beautiful You* journal, consider what surprised you about the film. How will what you learned influence your thoughts and actions moving forward?

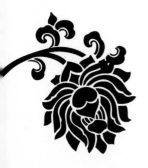

— 69 —

Ditch What Doesn't Fit

Y ou know the scene: It's Monday morning in your closet and you are desperately trying to put together something that fits (forget about mixing in a bit of your own personal style). Before you know it, fifteen minutes have passed and now you don't have time to finish anything else you need to do to get ready for work or school. Frustrated, you leave the house cranky—with chinks in your self-esteem and body-image armor.

Today —— Put aside some time to really go through your closet. Go through it item by item. Try things on that you haven't worn in awhile; make sure that tops have bottoms that match them; decide what fits and doesn't fit, as well as what you still like. Sort, sort, sort on your bed while you go. There should be a "Can Wear Now" pile, a "Want to Wear One Day" pile, and a "Give Away" pile.

Only the items in the "Can Wear Now" pile should find their way back into your closet. Go through your "Want to Wear One Day" pile one more time and keep only the items that really reflect you and your personal style—pieces that are truly irreplaceable. Store your "Want to Wear One Day" pile in an old suitcase or a plastic tub. Now run your "Give Away" pile to a local thrift store.

Back home, appreciate your clean closet and how it will allow you to get dressed more efficiently and more kindly every morning. Finally, make note of what you still need in your wardrobe (Black slacks? Brown kitten heels? Jeans to wear with flats?) and put that list in your handbag so that your shopping can be focused and intentional.

— 70 —

Get Some Perspective

One morning, I was eating my bowl of oatmeal while cruising the internet, and I came across a story about Halle Berry on the *Entertainment Tonight* site.

The sexy Halle Berry says she seeks the on-screen confidence of another actress! "Kate Winslet is always naked, sitting on a toilet, running buck-naked. She's free. I want to be the kind of actress who can really be comfortable with my body like that," she tells *Elle* magazine.

A few minutes later, I came across an article on Kate Winslet on the *Us Weekly* site.

Kate Winslet says she didn't always want to be famous. "I was fat. I didn't know any fat famous actresses," she tells December's *Vanity Fair.* "I just did not see myself in that world at all, and I'm being very sincere. You know, once a fat kid, always a fat kid," she adds. "Because you always think that you just look a little bit wrong or a little bit different from everyone else. And I still sort of have that."

Today ⸺ Go through your day believing that you—as you are right now—are fabulous. We spend so much time admiring the way other women look, and we do it in a way that's self-deprecating. The irony is that each woman we look at is doing the exact same thing—she's admiring the way some *other* woman looks. It's too much, really, this job we do on ourselves. We tell ourselves we're not enough—not pretty enough, nice enough, good enough, whatever enough. It is not our bodies that need to change. It's our minds.

— 71 —

Reconsider

You have been on this journey now for a couple months. Today we will reconsider what is standing in the way of our happiness, our brilliance.

Today ⟶ Answer this question in your *Beautiful You* journal: What holds you back?

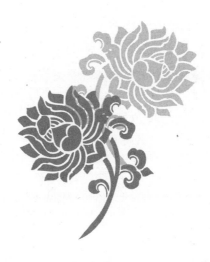

— 72 —

Stop Weighing Yourself

When a dear friend was two pounds away from her weight goal (she was perfectly healthy the way she was), she became obsessed with weighing herself. In the morning she'd weigh herself. After her run she'd weigh herself. Later, she'd weigh herself to see how food and water she'd taken in that day was affecting her weight. It was a vicious competition with the scale, and to her, the scale kept winning. Moreover, the battle with the scale didn't end with each weigh-in. It consumed her all day long. The scale still hadn't showed her the magical number, so it was broth for lunch. The scale was still being stingy, so it was lettuce for dinner. She was just two pounds away from her magic number, but her life was anything but majestic.

"Why don't you put away the scale and just go with how you feel?" I said.

It was like I'd asked her to kill her mother. But soon she began to see that the scale was both consuming her and haunting everything she consumed. She stopped weighing herself so often and learned to embrace the person she already was.

Today —— Step away from the scale. Do not give a little number on a little box on the middle of a floor somewhere in your house the power to dictate how you feel about yourself. Let your outlook be your guide. Choose an amount of time that seems challenging, and for that period, stop weighing yourself and focus instead on how your body feels.

Use Something You've Been Saving for a Special Occasion

I have this handbag that I love. It's a piece of art—silk birds set in patches of fabric in tropical colors—that just makes my heart sing. And because it is so beautiful, I never ever use it. It sits in my closet in a protective bag so that not even the dust can enjoy it. When I was young, my family couldn't afford nice things, and now I have a fear of the few nice things I do have. My husband gave me a beautiful necklace that I never wear because it's nice. You get the picture. I am terrified that by enjoying something, I'll ruin it, and so I don't enjoy it. I forget about it. But by not taking pleasure in the things I have, I deny myself delight. And being delighted is an essential part of well-being.

Today —— Use something that you've been saving for a special occasion and deliberately delight in it.

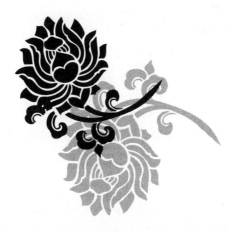

Drink Plenty of Water

It seems too simple to be true. But drinking plenty of water each day has a dramatic effect on your sense of well-being. When you are properly hydrated, you have more energy, better concentration, and more control over your moods. Poor hydration affects performance, causes tiredness and headaches, and reduces one's ability to concentrate and remain alert. Feeling our best really helps us be our best, and sometimes feeling better can be as simple as drinking more water.

Today — Drink more than enough water. Fill up a water bottle and keep it with you wherever you are. Challenge yourself to take sips throughout the day.

— 75 —

Look Up When You Walk

It was January in Roxbury, a Boston neighborhood where graffiti and gangs were the neighborhood norms. I was a junior in college, spending the last weeks of my winter break learning about youth violence and gang intervention programs in the area.

I had a rental car that I drove to the youth center each morning, and one afternoon, the sweet young men that I had come to know—they looked like typical gangbangers to others—watched as I left the building and worked my way down the gray street to my car.

"You all by yourself?" one of them called out.

Before I could answer, another one said, "Man, have you seen that girl walk? Ain't no one going to take her for a fool."

Years later, I remember this conversation most every time I am walking down an unfamiliar road or through an unfamiliar place. My face is lifted, my shoulders back, my smile ready, my eyes alert. I greet people as I walk past them. I signal that I belong wherever I end up.

Those young men in Roxbury taught me a simple but important lesson that day. We communicate so much without even saying a word. Strangers can surmise how we feel about ourselves—and how we feel about them— just by the way we hold ourselves as we walk by them. Carrying myself with an openness and awareness is just one way that I express the confidence I have in myself.

Today —— Look up when you walk. From your house to your car, your parking space to the office, across campus for class—wherever you are going, resist the urge to look down at the sidewalk or at your cell phone or iPod. Instead, engage in the world around you. Look around; see and allow yourself, no matter how difficult it is, to be seen. By the end of the day, you'll see the benefits you have reaped by taking the world in as you go, and your confidence in engaging other people, even nonverbally, will have increased.

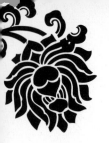

— 76 —

Take Three Ten-Minute Walks

Sometimes our confidence wavers because we feel so disconnected from our whole selves. We're out of touch with our body and our mind, and we're just going, going, going or doing, doing, doing. Today we're looking to bring some grounding to that going and doing.

Today —— Take three ten-minute walks. In the morning, plan when you'll take each walk, and then keep that commitment to yourself. As each walk unfolds, feel your muscles coming alive in the movement and just enjoy that feeling. Next, let your mind wander and see where it takes you.

At the end of the day, in your *Beautiful You* journal, reflect on the three walks: how they were different from each other, how you felt at the beginning and end of each one, what you learned and what you experienced.

Let Someone Know She Made A Difference

Speaking up about positive things people do is just as important as giving voice to your opinion about negative actions or situations. By bringing attention to things that are positive, encouraging, and hopeful, we are letting someone know she's done well and are encouraging more of that behavior in the future.

Today —— Let someone know she made a difference by acknowledging that her choices, decisions, and actions mattered—and that you noticed. By encouraging the good in this world, we create more good.

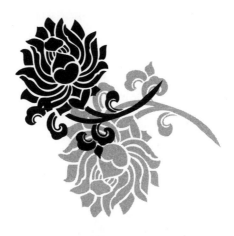

— 78 —

Eat Mindfully

W hat did you have for lunch?" someone might ask you, and you find yourself drawing a blank. Surely you had something, but why can't you think of it?

How many of us swallow our meals in two bites between meetings, in the front seat while carpooling, or standing in the kitchen while checking our Blackberry and talking to our spouses? Are most of our meals mere pit stops on the way to the rest of our lives or are they events in themselves, with their own opportunities for pleasure and reflection? For so much of the world, a meal is a gift, an act of reverence and nurturance. For too many of us, though, a meal is a race, a hassle, an inconvenience. When we reduce our sustenance to happenstance, we lose our attachment to being healthy, to honoring life, to connecting.

Today ⟶ Take the time to eat one of your meals mindfully. Set the table, sit down, savor the sensations of the meal, take small bites and sips of water. Enjoy the process. Enjoy not just the symbolism of it, but the truth behind it: you are nurturing your body and giving it fuel for that which is to come. By treating yourself well in this moment, you remind yourself of the value of treating yourself well in all moments.

— 79 —

Consider Your Needs

When I teach journaling, the content may change from workshop to workshop, but there is always one question that I keep because of its revelatory nature. "What," I ask my students, "do you need right now more than anything else?"

Not only do I ask my attendees to answer the question that day, I ask them to answer the question every day for seven days straight.

"Why seven days?" I am inevitably asked.

Because over seven days, you have a chance to compare your responses. It's one thing to have the same answer to the question two days in a row. But if you still have the same answer on day three, then the real question becomes this: Why don't you respect yourself enough to give yourself what you most need?

Today —— Answer this question in one to two sentences in your *Beautiful You* journal: What do I need right now more than anything else? Then figure out how to give it to yourself. Continue to ask yourself this question every day for the next week and monitor whether or not you are responding to your own needs.

— 80 —

Find Your Word

In my mid-twenties, I was at a conference for college administrators. We were asked to come up with one word that described our mission and follow that with a sentence that explained it.

"Voice," I said. It was my first succinct explanation of what I was finding to be my vocation.

What was my point in life? *To help people get at their own voices so they could express themselves and act from an authentic place.* Sometimes I could instigate that by using my own voice. Often times, I accomplished my mission by listening, questioning, suggesting.

Focusing on that one word ultimately led me to my mission statement. Having a mission statement helps me determine where and how I should and shouldn't be investing my time. Once you know your mission (we'll work on that later), you can find your way. It all starts with finding your word.

Today —— Stop right now and think about the one word that best describes what you are about, what your mission is in life. What comes to mind? Include your word in your *Beautiful You* journal.

— 81 —

Realize That Emotions Serve Us

So much of our unhealthy behavior stems from an emotional place. When we feel a negative emotion intensely, we often don't want to sit in it. We are scared of it, scared it might make us cry or sigh or bitch or moan or feel in some other way. We want it to go away. So we do things that will make it go away. We binge on food or alcohol or other substances that are bad for our bodies. We pick fights; we blame; we brood; we punish; we take it out on our bodies. But emotions are not there to punish us. They are there to serve us, to give us information, to help us gather insight, to teach us. In fact, a University of Missouri study revealed that negative feelings can actually yield greater happiness in the long term because those negative feelings show us what needs to be reassessed. Learning from our pasts, after all, can help us plan a better future.

Today —— Allow yourself to feel what you feel. Don't look to stuff your emotion, feed it, quiet it, or squelch it. Instead, just be with it. Allow it to teach you what it was meant to teach you. Allow yourself to learn what you are meant to learn.

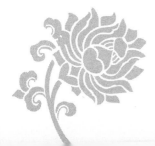

DAY

— 82 —

Don't Listen to the One

I was driving an eighth-grade girl I know home from lunch. We were passing by the university where I teach, and I pointed it out to her.

"What do you teach?" she asked, and I explained what Women and Gender Studies was and, more specifically, what body image was.

"Like how I think I'm fat?" she asked, when I finished explaining that we spend the semester considering how individuals feel about their bodies and looks, what causes those feelings, and how they can be addressed.

My heart stopped. "How long have you thought you were fat?" I asked.

"Since last year."

"Did something happen to make you think that?"

"Yes," she said. " My friend, who is really skinny—and skinnier than I would want to be—told me I was too heavy."

"And since she told you that, how many people have told you that you were beautiful?"

She looked at me, confused as to what one thing had to do with the other. "I don't know. A lot, I guess."

"Have you been told that probably a hundred times in the last year?"

"I guess so. Yes."

"When that girl said you were too heavy, that statement was a lot more about her than it was about you," I said. "For whatever reason, she is insecure, and she deals with it by pointing out things to other people who might fuel her insecurity. Does that make sense?"

She looked at me and nodded, and slowly began to relay things she had observed in her friend that might reveal the depth of her insecurities.

"Why listen to this one person?" I told her. "Why let her opinion have so much weight, especially given what you've been told by so many other people and given what you thought about yourself—that you were just fine—up until the day this one friend said that to you?"

"That's a very good question," she answered, and she looked out her window.

Today —— Think about the things you believe because just one person said them to you. Why listen to that one?

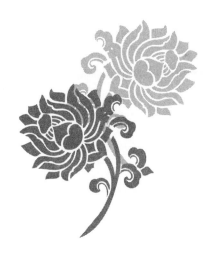

DAY

— 83 —

Talk Yourself Out of the Beauty Myth

Rationally, you already know plenty of reasons why you shouldn't buy into the beauty myth. That doesn't mean you don't buy into it, but it does mean you should remember how much you already know and what you already feel deep down inside.

Today —— In your *Beautiful You* journal, write down all the reasons you should stop obsessing over your appearance. Remind yourself of these insights whenever you are blindsided by body brooding.

— 84 —

Understand That Your Choices Are Yours Alone

H ere's the deal. Someone is always going to be unhappy with the decisions you make. Someone is always going to love them. You just can't play to your audience—as much as you want to be the good girl, as much as you want people to like you, even as much as you want to do the right thing. The only right thing to do is to do what you want most, to act in a way that contributes to your overall well-being and supports your best intentions, given who you are and where you are now. Your happiness is yours for the choosing. Becoming comfortable enough to make the choices you want and need means becoming confident enough to act from an authentic place.

Today —— Understand that every single choice you make today—and everyday—is yours alone. Go forward making choices that do not allow the noise around you to change what is true for you.

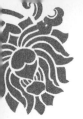

— 85 —

Enjoy Some Body Work

I was an overworked and exhausted second-year teacher and coach when I scheduled my first massage. It was a Thursday, and every muscle in my body ached. I was sitting in my classroom during a planning period, thinking about how I might make it to the soccer game I needed to coach that night, when my hands, almost with their own agenda, reached over to the phone book on my desk and started combing the *Yellow Pages* for spas. I found one that wasn't too far from the school and called to see if they could squeeze me in after school let out, before I needed to be back for the game. They fit me in, and that hour was so restorative that I physically ran the drills with the team as they warmed up that night. Now massage is a regular feature of my self-care regimen, and I encourage you to make it a part of yours too. A study done by the University of Miami School of Medicine's Touch Research Institute revealed that getting a thirty-minute massage regularly—for example, one every other week—can boost overall body satisfaction, no matter your shape or size.

Today ⟿ Schedule a massage. If it's too expensive for your budget, consider asking for a gift certificate as a gift, booking a thirty-minute session instead of a one-hour one, or calling a local massage school to ask about their practice sessions, which can cost one-third of the price of a regular massage. Or check out your local Whole Foods to see if they offer inexpensive chair massages.

Watch *Real Women Have Curves*

One way to expand our perspective of ourselves is to broaden the images and stories we see and hear about women. While many films categorize women in narrow or negative ways, others are expansive.

Today —— Borrow and watch *Real Women Have Curves*. Set in Los Angeles, *Real Women Have Curves* follows Ana, a Mexican-American teenager struggling to break free from the expectations her mother has for her. You'll stand up and cheer during one especially memorable sewing shop scene, and maybe even take a little bit of Ana's gumption with you into your day.

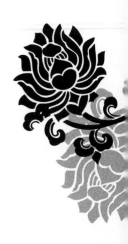

— 87 —

Make a "Caught You" Box

Working on our own self-esteem is tough. Helping our children develop positive self-esteem can feel even more challenging. But when you are young, nothing feels better than having your parents notice what you've done right. Use that human need to be recognized to your advantage to help your children bask in their brilliance.

Today —— Have children? Create a "Caught You" box and put it in a place of prominence in your home. Store note cards and pens inside. When you catch someone in your family doing something that makes you feel proud of him or her, write it on a note card and place it in the box. Encourage everyone else in your family to do the same. Once a week, open up the "Caught You" box when the family is all gathered together and take turns reading the accolades out loud.

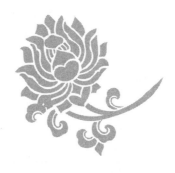

DAY

—— 88 ——

Picture Yourself Fulfilled

The picture captures me as a first-year teacher and coach, age 23. In it, I am lying across desks in my classroom, dressed for coaching that afternoon's soccer game. My cheeks are pressed into round apples, my mouth is pulled into a joker-like grin, my teeth are biting the tip of my tongue—it's the quirky thing I do with my smile when I'm at my most joyful. My hair is pulled tightly back in a ponytail, but you can still see what inspired my student to take this picture—I've dyed my raven hair royal blue to celebrate our team's first win of the season. If I could choose just one picture to show what teaching and coaching meant to me, it would be this one. The joy, purpose, and passion I felt in that work is captured in that dye job, that smile, that lack of self-consciousness. Being reminded of this young woman is like a bridge to my best self, and that is why this picture stays on my desk, even when other things come and go. It's a flash of my core, a touchstone that's always present, just in case I need a reminder when I am not feeling like myself.

Today —— Find a photo from one of the most joyful times in your life, a time when you were content and self-satisfied—even if it's when you were six—and place it somewhere you will see it often and be reminded of your best, most joyful self. When you are feeling down about where you are or the way you look, track your eyes over to that photo for a reminder that you have been to that place of joy and fulfillment, and that you can return.

— 89 —

Focus on Your Best Feature

It's a Friday night, the baby's in bed, and the perfect way for me to relax is with the newest episode of *What Not to Wear*. While I love Clinton Kelly and Stacy London's funny banter and good advice, my favorite part is when the makeover recipient lands in Carmindy's makeup chair.

"What do you see when you look in the mirror?" she always asks.

The answers go something like this: "Red, splotchy skin." "Bags under my eyes." "Wrinkles." You get the picture.

Then there is Carmindy's refreshing but clear reaction.

"When I look in that mirror, I see great skin, amazing green eyes, and a lovely smile."

Carmindy gives each makeover recipient what we all need. She sees a woman's best feature, celebrates it, and then says, "Let's make everyone notice it."

We each have that unique thing about us that draws someone's eye when they look at our face, but we forget about it far too often when we distract ourselves in the mirror with what we don't like.

Today —— Consider your best feature. Is it your big, brown eyes, your smile that lights up the room, or those sweet freckles you've had since you were a girl? What makes your face distinctly unique? For today, style your hair or put on makeup (if you use it) it in a way that highlights your best feature. Then bask in the beauty that is uniquely your own.

Quit Dating

I fell in love with teaching from the start. While that love and passion was developing, the relationship I was in, one that had lasted years, was slowly drawing to a close. It wasn't that we didn't love each other anymore, but we lived three states apart and neither of us knew where we would go next. He wanted an M.D., I was eyeing an M.F.A., and those programs would take us to new places that might ultimately lead us even further apart physically. And so, on a tearful night at the end of a wonderful week together, we said good-bye.

Not long after, I thought about dating again. It seemed an easy way to get rid of the wound my heart had suffered, a benign way to self-medicate the pain of lost love. But I knew that dating again would be the easy way out of grieving the loss and, even more importantly, an avoidance of getting to know who I was becoming at that time in my life. Instead, I decided to do something really different. I decided that I would not date seriously for a year. When I was asked out, I either said "no" or told the person right from the start that if he was looking for someone to go to a restaurant with that one time, I was the girl. If he was looking for a possible relationship, I wasn't.

That year helped me really get to know myself and understand what it was I could provide for myself and what I really wanted in a relationship; it showed me that I would be just fine.

Today —— If you are single and in a chronic pattern of dating people who aren't right for you, it's likely because you don't *know* what's right for you. Decide right now to take some time off from dating or even being intimate with someone. It doesn't have to be a year. It can be three months. But make it deliberate. Give yourself a chance to get to know the person you are right now, and the truth of what it is you want for yourself, without the filter of a relationship that you force to make work in spite of yourself.

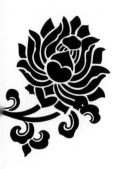

Create a Soundtrack

There are some really great female empowerment songs out there. These are songs that celebrate womanhood in all its glory—without calling for a partner to do the rescuing. These are songs that say "*I can rescue me.*" They make no mention of a man coming in and making things better, and they are all about embracing female power. Sometimes we need that soundtrack playing in the background (or foreground) of our lives while we do what we must do.

Today —— Create your own "I Can Rescue Me" playlist. Have it ready to blast at a minute's notice when you need some strong music to back you up. And, if you're game, come share it at www.rosiemolinary.com so that other readers can glean from your suggestions.

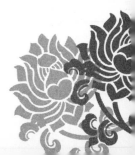

— 92 —

Learn How to Look Great in a Photo

I was watching an *America's Next Top Model* marathon when I noticed that textbook good looks don't automatically make a great photo. As it turns out, there is a science to a great photo that has nothing to do with whether or not you are 5'1" or 5'10", blonde or brunette, etc. The truth behind my suspicion was confirmed when I went to have pictures taken by a photographer. I was miserable about having my photo taken, but a magazine that was featuring me required it. I always look like a deer in headlights in photos and expected the worst from the proofs. When I saw them, though, I was pleasantly surprised. It wasn't that suddenly, between waking up that morning and driving to the photographer's house, I'd become a runway model. It was that she knew how to talk me through the photo shoot in a way that delivered photos that really captured my essence. And we all know that a good photo is a great boost to one's self-confidence.

Today —— Have someone take a photograph of you, and pose just as you normally would. Now have him or her take a photo while you follow these tips, which I have learned from various photographers. First, bend your arms at least a little bit to create some space between your body and your arms. Put a hand on your waist or put your hands in the front pockets of a long sweater with a slight bend in your elbow. Next, make sure the photographer is slightly higher than you are; he or she should be pointing the camera down. Then turn your face slightly to the side, so you aren't looking at the camera head on (avoid my deer in headlights look!). Finally, don't smile as soon as the camera appears—your smile will just fade away by the time the photo is snapped. Just before the picture is taken, laugh softly out loud and you'll get a natural smile.

— 93 —

Don't Be a Consumer

Sometimes, when we are emotionally starved, we are inclined to think that consumption will fulfill us. That consumption can be food, but most often, it's *stuff*. We search for the perfect lip gloss as if we are on the road to the Holy Grail. We think that new boots will complete us. We look for meaning in our stuff. But unless we are being deliberate, we rarely find it.

Today —— Do not buy anything. Instead, use what you have and spend time reflecting on where you are in life. If it's hard for you, write a list of your needs in your *Beautiful You* journal, don't buy anything, and revisit that list in a week to see if the items on your list are still legitimate needs.

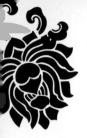

Choose Happiness

Ever met someone who was handling a very difficult circumstance with grace, gratitude, and joy? I have, and I've walked away from my exchanges with the person thinking, "I don't know if I could ever handle it that well." The lesson is that intention is a powerful thing, and we can choose to deliberately enjoy life, even when it's hard. Because the truth is, most of life is not only out of *our* control, but out of control, period. What we do have the power to do is choose happiness.

Today —— Choose happiness. Make decisions all day long that allow you to experience happiness, even in the face of something tougher.

Look at Yourself Differently

I n our woeful laments, we call them wrinkles—those expression lines that creep up beside our eyes, on our forehead, or around our mouths. But what those lines really show is the life we have lived and the way that we have experienced it.

Today —— Look at yourself differently. Experience your crow's feet as signs of your smiling joy. Your laugh lines as signs that you have laughed heartily in your life. Your forehead lines as symbols of your expressive self. The life you have lived to earn each one of those expression lines has been earnest and true. All they show is the joy and care and love that you have had in your heart, your willingness to feel your way through life. That's not something to be criticized or lamented. It is something to be celebrated.

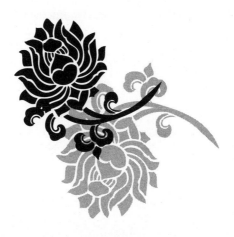

— 96 —

Consider Your Goals

Growing up, we're told over and over again that life is not just about the money we make, the things we have, the attention we get, or our looks. We want to believe it, but sometimes, maybe, we wonder if perhaps those things really could make us happy—or at least make our lives a bit easier.

Not so much, say three University of Rochester researchers whose report on the subject was published in the June 2009 issue of the *Journal of Research in Personality*. The researchers studied recent college graduates and assessed their state of well-being after the young people had achieved goals they had set for themselves.

They found that the more committed an individual is to a goal, the greater her likelihood of achieving it. But that doesn't necessarily mean that her success will make her happy. In fact, researchers found that reaching materialistic and image-related goals actually contributed to more negative feelings, such as shame and anger, and more symptoms of anxiety. Meanwhile, achieving goals related to personal growth, relationships, community involvement, and physical health led to a greater sense of satisfaction, happiness, well-being, and a more positive sense of self. Well-being, it turns out, is really about meeting one's basic needs for autonomy, competence, and relatedness through connecting with what's inside rather than outside.

Today —— Consider what the researchers found. In your *Beautiful You* journal, reflect on your personal goals and identify which ones are driven by your desire for personal growth, better relationships, more meaningful community involvement, and greater wellness. Which ones are motivated by other desires? How can you tweak your goals in a way that meets your needs for personal growth?

Keep a Master List of Joys

There are moments in my life that I continue to delight in, long after the experiences have passed. As I get older, more memories are added to the fold, but sometimes I remember past experiences a little less crisply. Realizing this, I decided to start journaling for my son every Sunday, writing down everything that brought us joy that week so that it will always be with us. That practice has made me want to capture other joyful experiences as well. I find that they renew my spirit, remind me of my essence, and give me a sense of well-being.

Today ⬎— Designate the last fifteen pages in your *Beautiful You* journal as your "Joy Pages." On the first sheet, today, write down a list of moments you have had in your life that just delighted you. In the days to come, write a paragraph about each moment, capturing everything that makes your heart feel lighter because of that experience.

— 98 —

Celebrate Yourself

Sometimes we forget to cherish the beauty of who we are. Today, we will do just that.

Today —— Open your *Beautiful You* journal, and complete this sentence by celebrating your sterling attributes.

I am . . .

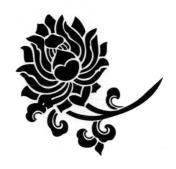

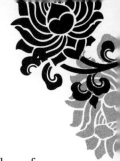

DAY

— 99 —

Go Big

"**H**ere comes one," my partner says, and my eyes flicker to the surf.

Out of the water, a 700-pound leatherback turtle, one of the oldest animals on this planet and one of just a few thousand still alive, struggles to pull herself across the sand. She looks prehistoric as she moves forward with deliberate, heavy steps. She is following the call of her genetic code, returning to the beach where she was born to lay her own eggs. We are here to meet her, to record her visit for science, to see if we can help change the count.

She finds a place to nest and uses her back limbs like shovels. When the digging stops, she enters a trance that will last the entire time she lays her billiard-ball sized eggs. We inspect her, measure her, tag her back limbs, and microchip her shoulder. She lays almost one hundred eggs, filling the nest, and then covers it with a series of frenzied strokes to camouflage the nest from predators.

She turns back toward the ocean, her heavy body lunging forward. This is the part that overwhelms me, that makes me realize the amazing thing that I have just witnessed—nature trying to beat the odds—and I tear up. But it is more than nature beating the odds that overwhelms me in this moment. I am moved, too, by just how small I am. By how inconsequential my worries can be. By remembering that there is so much that matters more than my thighs or hair or waist size. There, in the pitch black night of Trinidad's Matura beach, I experience one of those moments where my smallness, both figuratively and literally, implants itself in me, reminding me of what matters, reminding me of why I matter.

Today —— Go somewhere—to a vast field, a rock quarry, a mountain path, an ocean front—that allows you to feel small. Perch there. Compare your obsessions to the vastness in front of you and gain perspective.

⟶ 100 ⟶

Realize That You Are the One Who Cares Most

One of my students recently told me she spent a good part of the previous few months losing the eight pounds she had gained during the summer. Finally at her goal weight, she felt satisfied and proud.

At a recent dinner, Erin shared her accomplishment with her family and boyfriend. Everyone looked at her with surprise, unaware that she had lost any weight. Watching their faces, she realized in a rush that she was the only one who had noticed and cared about her weight gain (or her weight loss).

"Everyone is so busy with their own issues, problems, and busy life that they don't have the energy to worry about what other people's bodies look like or how much others weigh" she said. "I was creating my own misery and stress. . . . I thought that by being skinny I would be noticed and accepted, when the reality is that it was all very trivial to everyone else except me."

Today ⟶ Realize that you are the one who cares most about the standards you have created. You are your toughest judge. Release yourself from those impossibly high standards, which only lead you to unhappiness, and you release yourself into the possibility of greater self-satisfaction and fulfillment.

— 101 —

Imagine That Nothing Changes

So often, we live our lives with the assumption that our bodies, our looks, will change one day and that when that day comes, we can give ourselves more permission to enjoy life. We say, "If only I had (insert your running commentary here—a flatter stomach, bigger boobs, a more delicate nose, straighter hair), then everything in my life would be right. Everything would change." But what if that doesn't happen?

Today —— Imagine that nothing changes—that how you look today is how you will look for the rest of your life. Your weight never changes; your hair never grows; your teeth are never bleached. In your *Beautiful You* journal, reflect on these questions. If you were to live out the rest of your life just as you are today, what would you want to make sure you got to do? How would you live if this were it? What would you do different than you do today? Start living that way now.

— 102 —

Remember That Your Body Is a Blessing

During my weekly body-image seminar, we always take a break halfway through the three-hour class. Once, in the middle of our break, one of my students approached me.

"I just got a message that my brother had a seizure and is in the hospital. Do you mind if I go?"

"Absolutely not," I answered, and then I expressed concern for her brother.

As we talked a little more, I asked if he had ever had a seizure before. She told me he suffered from a chronic illness that had taken a turn for the worse, and they weren't sure how things were going to turn out for him. As she ran out of class, another student, who sits near the front of my classroom, looked up at me.

"Well that just makes all of this stuff," she motioned around the room with her hands, indicating the body obsession and beauty standards we speak of so often in class, "seem petty now, doesn't it?"

I nodded at her and said, "Our bodies are really amazing gifts, if we would only see that. We spend so much time belittling the small things that we miss the big picture all together."

Today —— Remember that your body is a blessing.

— 103 —

Stock the Pantry

Part of embracing the wholeness of your beauty is moving past it, to see the expanse of the world and its needs. Today our efforts concentrate on getting out of ourselves and into some of the important work of the world. When we see ourselves doing something that really matters, we see our whole selves—beautiful, committed, loving.

Today —— Call or visit your local food bank's website to find out what it needs most and then pay a visit to the grocery store. After you stock up on much-needed staples, drop them off at the food bank and bask in the beauty of investing in the lives of your neighbors.

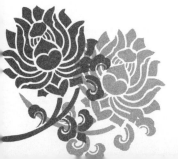

— 104 —

Look at the World with Your Smallest Eye

We can name the smallest flaw that we think exists on our face. We can be nitpicky about our hair texture until we have put another person to sleep. We notice *everything* about ourselves in our quest for improvement or perfection, and yet we rarely use that same careful, observant eye when we're looking at the world.

Today —— Take your camera with you wherever you go and look at your world with that smallest of eyes—with your camera's zoom lens. Everywhere you go, snap pictures of the details around you. By forcing yourself to use your exacting eyes to see the world, rather than critique your face, you open yourself up to the variety that naturally exists in our surroundings and the beauty that is present in all its nuances.

— 105 —

Watch What You Say

In the seminar I teach, we look at the way parents and peers have an impact on one's body image. I wish I could say I have to struggle to find examples to share with the class each semester. But in fact, I don't bother coming up with examples at all before class because every semester my students have plenty.

They tell the stories you'd expect: How their mother's chronic talk of needing to lose weight made them self-conscious about their bodies, how their father's comments about someone's looks impacted what they saw as beautiful, how their older sister's strict dieting made them swear off carbs forever. Words that seem harmless can actually create an unrealistic expectation about looks and behavior. Our negative talk, as it turns out, can actually be contagious.

Today — You have been working on avoiding negative talk about your appearance for a while now. The question is, How are you doing—especially in front of the children in your life? Watch every word that you say in front of your daughters, nieces, and girls you mentor, and make sure you avoid negative statements about looks, food, weight, body size, and shape. Girls pay more attention to what we do and say than we realize, and what we say shapes their body image.

— 106 —

Learn Your Lesson

Just as we are not our looks, we are also not the things that happen to us. Too often, we take less-than-perfect things that occur in our lives—many of which we have no control over—and give them negative meanings they are not meant to have. Instead, they can simply be teaching moments, experiences that put us on a journey of further understanding and awareness.

Today —— In your *Beautiful You* journal, write down two to four difficult experiences or losses that you have experienced in your life. Next to each experience or loss, reflect on what lesson you learned from it and what you gained from the experience. How are you wiser now for having gone through that experience? Walk away from this exercise knowing that we are not the things that happen to us. We are, instead, a compilation of what we learn and how we are in the world.

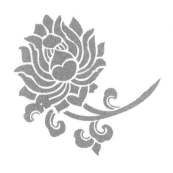

— 107 —

Reflect on Your Desired Tributes

None of us goes through life with just one role. We are each someone's child, maybe someone's sister, possibly a mother, a student, an employee, a teacher, a coach, an athlete, a spouse or partner. We might be a Christian, a Jew, a Buddhist, a Muslim, a Hindu. Perhaps we embrace our role as a feminist, a Republican, a Democrat, a Latina, an African-American, a Native American, an Indian. The list of potential roles we play in our lives goes on and on. The reality, too, is that we are not the same person in each role that we play. There are different nuances to our roles, different ways we need to be supportive in them, different ways we need to accomplish what we need to get done. By embracing our roles and being fully who we need to be in each one, we gain valuable confidence.

Today ⟞ In your *Beautiful You* journal, list the roles you play in your life. Next to each one, write a one- to three-sentence tribute you would like to receive, based on how you act in that role. Are you there yet? What do you need to do to embody who you fully wish to be in every role you play?

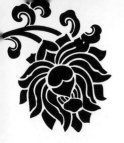

— 108 —

Make the Right Decision

oo often, we concentrate on what we *wish* we looked like. We pour over magazine pages searching for the likeness we most wish to emulate. We gaze at television screens longingly. We eye our peers in envy, hope, despair. We spend so much time longing for a certain appearance that we let what is really essential fall from our priority list.

Today — Decide what you want to do with your life, not what you want to look like in this life, because it is what you do that will make an impact. It is what you *do* that will thrill you.

— 109 —

Get Clear on Your Intention

Knowing what you want out of life is the first step to making plans and making certain you are on track. But it is important to pick goals that are derived from your own desires, not those that are influenced by others. Once you know what it is you want, you can move towards it with clarity, conviction, and purpose.

Today —— Get clear on your intention. Consider what you want for your life in your *Beautiful You* journal. Where are you on your journey to making your intention a reality? What attitude do you need to have for this journey? What skills do you need to practice or obtain? Knowing that you are on a journey that is your own and moving forward deliberately allows you to feel the reward of every moment of progress.

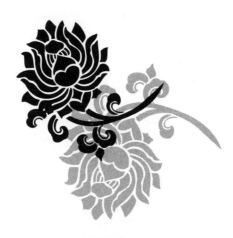

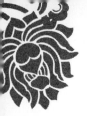

— 110 —

Design Your Life

Part of our unhappiness with ourselves can be rooted in an incongruence between what we want for ourselves and what we are actually allowing for ourselves. By more deliberately claiming what we want, we move toward greater satisfaction.

Today — Answer these questions in your *Beautiful You* journal. What would your ideal life be like? What would each day look like? Who would you share it with? Next, consider what you must do to get there. Write down some steps to help you move toward your ideal life. Every day, take one step that moves you closer to your truth.

— 111 —

Reflect on Where Your Time and Energy Go

"There aren't enough hours in a day."

How many of us have been there, said that? Not only are there not enough hours in the day, but there isn't enough energy for everything we are asked to do or expect ourselves to do. By reviewing where we put our time and energy, we become better aware and learn to prioritize the finite amount of time and energy we have for the experiences that are most important to us.

Today ⟶ In your *Beautiful You* journal, write down how you spent your time over the last five days. Next, consider where your energy goes, but not just your physical energy. Also consider your mental energy, your emotional energy, your creative energy, and your spiritual energy. Now look over your notes. Which energy uses drain you rather than replenish you? Which time commitments take away from your world rather than add to it?

— 112 —

Name Your Priorities

I n order to be the best version of our selves, it is important that we devote our time and energy to things that are truly important to us. When we give our time away to things that do not hold much meaning for us, we begin to lose touch with the truest version of ourselves; we find ourselves having to fake it. Losing touch with our truest self carries us away, rather than toward, our self-esteem.

Today —— In your *Beautiful You* journal, name your priorities. What activities in your life do you most value? Which offer you benefits that equal the amount of energy you put into them? What people do you want to make sure have a regular place in your life? By naming your priorities, you can begin to deliberately embrace them, adding more purpose and passion to your life.

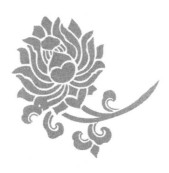

DAY

— 113 —

Say No

I lose my way most quickly when I enter a period of saying yes too often. In periods where my calendar is over-scheduled, I feel off center. My work suffers. My family suffers. The truth is, I suffer. By studying my calendar and my own rhythms, I now know that there are times I should never make appointments.

While I know my priorities, I still lose my way sometimes and say yes to something I shouldn't have. When I lose my focus and lose my center, I lose my sense of self. And losing your sense of self, even temporarily, can really rattle your confidence. While declining an invitation or refusing a commitment isn't always easy, living with what you said yes to can sometimes be even harder. Keeping that in mind has helped me gather more resolve.

Today —— When I have to say no, I always worry that I will disappoint someone. But I have found instead that people are usually far less attached to you doing something than you think they will be. Often when I say no, they forget it and simply move on.

Today, when you are asked anything—Want to go to lunch? Can you make a cake for the office party?—resist the urge to automatically say yes. Instead, think about it. Ask yourself if you would enjoy this commitment or if you would be doing it out of obligation. Then respond appropriately.

I usually couch my "no" responses in language that shows that the issue for me is bigger than that one thing. For example, I'll say, "Thank you so much for thinking of me. I have made a commitment to myself (and/or my family) and I just can't add anything to my plate right now. I am so sorry to have to say no to this opportunity, but I know that you will find just the right person for it." After some practice saying no and realizing that others are more understanding than you thought they would be, it becomes easier to protect your time, and you'll be able to apply that saved energy and effort to your own needs and interests.

DAY

— 114 —

Let Go

W e've talked about saying no to new invitations, but if you're anything like me, even after I feel resolve, my calendar still has commitments I wish I hadn't put there. What do we do about the ways we have already filled up our lives with things that aren't in sync with who we are or where we are going?

We bow out of them gracefully.

By bringing more balance to your life, you create the opportunity to actually enjoy, relish, and cherish everything you do choose to do. And when you can experience that joy—that bliss of being fulfilled in just the right way, by just the right situations, in just the right amount—you are more attuned to your truest self.

Today —— Look at your schedule for the next three months. What is on it that doesn't need to be? Go ahead and create space to breathe, to be, to dream—to become your truest self—by eliminating the things you truly do not have it in your heart to do.

— 115 —

Create an Internal Yardstick

oo often, we compare ourselves and our successes to other people. For a healthier self-image, consider your growth and achievement in light of who you are and where you have been.

Today —— In your *Beautiful You* journal, make a list of your achievements over the last year. These can include things nobody else noticed—such as how much you have learned at work over the past year, or how much more comfortable you are about public speaking.

Now think about the year ahead. What are some accomplishments you'd like to achieve? List those in your journal too. You are creating your own internal yardstick, something you can check-in with occasionally to measure your progress.

— 116 —

Compliment a Child in Your Life

We all remember a kind word that was said to us when we were children. In fact, many of us have held onto those childhood compliments, making sure that the trait illuminated by another person's words will always be a part of who we are. The value of a compliment in a child's life might just be immeasurable. When we take the time to notice their efforts, talents, accomplishments, and values, we teach children that the true value of a person is measured in their character, in how they live, in the way their values spring to life in action.

Today —— Pay a child or the children in your life a compliment. Help them understand what makes them special, and empower them to realize that any negativity they face in life isn't about them, but about the person saying those negative words.

— 117 —

Teach People How to Treat You

The first time it happened was on a cruise ship. We were seniors at different high schools, and our senior classes were taking graduation cruises together. He chose to go. I chose not to. But I made him a mixed tape so that he could have me there in spirit, one with great classic rock songs that would come back to bite me, like "Love the One You're With." It turns out he did (love the one he was with).

It seemed like a defining moment, and for my definition, I chose what I always had when it came to relationships: I was calm, rational, nice, and forgiving. If I broke up with him, I reasoned, then I would be allowing him to make me a different person—a vengeful, jealous person, and that's not who I was. So I called the girl he'd been with and said I wouldn't make things awkward, the issue was between me and him. I heard his teary pleas, challenged him, and said it would be hard to earn my trust again, but we could try.

A month later, I decided on a college. I had received an acceptance to the school where he'd enrolled, but I had no desire to follow a boy. I chose to go elsewhere, and we decided to see how a long-distance relationship worked. That summer, I found out he hadn't swapped spit with only one girl on that cruise. But since I had already forgiven him the one, how the hell could I hold this new *old* news against him? I fussed a bit; I made motions; and I stayed.

That fall it kept happening. He'd kiss one girl here, another there. It's what he did. What *I* did was figure out how to appear firm while still being nice. Meanwhile, my friends came to me with their troubles. I was a good listener, and I was always clear. "You deserve more," I would tell these women I loved. I wanted to see them honor their right to be fully cared for—by themselves and by whomever they let into their heart.

"We teach people how to treat us," I insisted, and yet it took months for those words to ring true in my own ears. There was a disconnect between the girl who championed others and the girl who couldn't champion herself. I finally learned that it wasn't enough to believe in the worth and dignity and rights of everyone else. I needed to offer myself that same justice. I called him one spring night and ended it.

There is never a day where it is better to be in a relationship that undermines, undercuts, manipulates, abuses, or takes advantage of us than it is to be single and in a relationship with ourselves that's filled with self-love. There is no man or woman worth the loss of our sense of dignity or selves. We must stop these relationships before they start. We can learn to trust our intuition, back away quickly, and teach and encourage others to do the same. Being good, it turns out, isn't about pleasing. Being good is about being just to others while also being true to yourself.

Today —— In your *Beautiful You* journal, reflect on your present and past relationships. Are there any that you get or got lost in? Write about the disconnect between what you need(ed) and what you receive(d) in those relationships and how it affects or affected you. Strategize about how you can use this knowledge to move forward and truthfully teach the people in your life how to treat you.

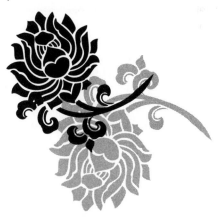

— 118 —

Invest in Someone Else

Sometimes we get so absorbed in our own world that we lose perspective. We become consumed by a bad haircut, acne, an uninspired wardrobe, or whatever else is plaguing us, and we lose sight of the world beyond us. Sometimes I think self-consciousness is almost a luxury, an extravagance we plague ourselves with when life isn't filling up our attention otherwise. But everywhere, every day, there are so many people who do not have the luxury of time or energy to become absorbed with a bad haircut (like I am right now) because their lives are faced with challenges that I will never know.

Microlending allows everyday citizens to make loans to entrepreneurs they don't necessarily know, loans that will help support a small business. Sponsoring organizations link lenders around the world to potential borrowers and facilitate these small loan transactions, as well as their repayment. When the entrepreneur pays back her loan to the sponsoring organization, the lender's investment is returned so that it can be reinvested or transferred back to her bank account.

Kiva is one of the organizations uniting people from around the world as lenders and entrepreneurs. On its website, www.Kiva.org, you can find photos of entrepreneurs, descriptions of their businesses, and plans for their loans, so you can see what types of efforts are supported. You can't always know which person or effort will receive your loan, but it will go to the country you select. Kiva partners with microfinance institutions in each participating country, so there is significant expertise in the field and assurance that investments are handled responsibly.

Sometimes it is helpful to get away from that little thing that is bothering us and take a look at something bigger.

Today ⤙ Visit www.Kiva.org or another micro-lending site and review the opportunities. Make a $25 investment in a country where the projects inspire you. Bookmark the page and periodically monitor—and cheer on— the effort's progress. Enjoy the satisfaction of having strengthened your connection to the world.

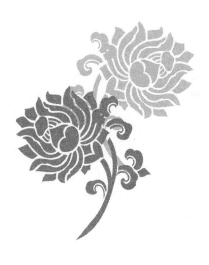

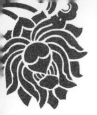

Have Faith

Polly Campbell, a blogger for *Psychology Today*, is a Portland, Oregon-based writer who specializes in issues of spirituality. Her faith and spiritual practice have had a significant impact on her ability to see herself more positively.

"Wayne Dyer once wrote a prayer that said, 'Thank you for all that I am and all that I have,' and it made such an impression on me," she says. "When I say that prayer, I am honoring the God, the universe, that created me. We are already intact. We already have much of what we need. I don't have to have it all figured out. I can trust that in my learning process, others will show up to coach me and, if not, an energy will be there to guide me. That is really useful on the days when you don't know how it's going to work out and even on the days that are really great."

Campbell is working on a book, *Imperfect Spirituality,* about how to integrate spiritual practices and self-improvement principles into our daily routines.

Today — Regardless of your spiritual history, begin the day by whispering Dyer's prayer and embracing the concept of faith. Each time doubt or worry enters your mind, give way to the notion that there is a force in the universe that will insure that things will work out. By practicing faith, you begin to hone your confidence and realize that you are just as you should be.

— 120 —

Realize That Life Keeps Handing You the Lesson You Need

I mentioned earlier that an old boyfriend cheated on me, and that I initially stayed with him. I wanted to be nice, to behave in a way I was most familiar with, so I stayed. But ultimately, he continued to be attracted to other women, and I realized that our own actions teach people how to treat us.

That big lesson wasn't the only one I learned from that experience. I also learned that life keeps handing you the lesson you need to learn until you learn it. Ignore the lesson, dismiss its significance, and the need to learn it won't go away. It will just come at you later, at an amplified volume, until you can no longer ignore it.

As my boyfriend kept cheating, I couldn't break up with him—not because I thought he was "the one" or that I needed to have a boyfriend, but because breaking up with someone went against my understanding of myself as a nice, sweet, easygoing girl. How can you be sweet and easygoing while breaking up with a guy for his own lack of sweetness, respect, and judgment? It seemed that forgiving him was much more in line with who I was, so I went there—until I realized that these moments between him and other women were lessons for both of us: We were not meant to be together. These incidents continued to happen because we weren't learning the lesson being provided to us. Life was amplifying the volume. We were missing the point.

Ever since that experience, I've tried my darnedest to learn my lessons early on—to prevent additional wounds I'll have to lick. Sometimes it works; I'm on the ready and hyper-vigilant. Sometimes, I am dense enough to miss it until the volume is at a crescendo. When that happens, I remind myself that while life can be a series of steps forward followed mercilessly by steps back—the setbacks aren't absolute unless I make them that way. The key is to get yourself tuned in, so when the pendulum swings you can bail before you lose all traction.

Today —— Consider what lessons life has been trying to teach you. Are you listening closely so that you can hear them before life cranks up the volume?

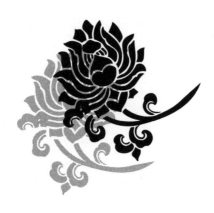

— 121 —

Realize It's Not About You

Here is what I have learned about the feedback people give us. Whether it is positive or negative, it's much more about the person giving it than it is about us. The person who tells you that you have a fabulous smile may be self-conscious about her own smile or her lack of joy. The person who tells you that you need to watch your weight is likely watching her own weight. Regardless of how much those comments might be about the person who says them, we tend to take them fairly seriously. I still remember that one of my ninth-grade teachers told me I needed to wear eyeliner (I kid you not). Seriously, what fourteen-year-old girl needs eyeliner so badly that you would tell her that in class? Not that many, right? So whatever the deal was with eyeliner for that teacher, the comment was much more about her than it was about me.

Today ——— Try not to take what other people say so seriously. Who cares what someone thinks about your hair, dress, lipstick, partner, or plans? Perhaps they're right, but it's just as likely they're wrong, and the only thing that matters is that you listen to what you want for yourself.

DAY

— 122 —

Refuse to Be a Billboard

We all have items in our wardrobes—things that have been given to us or we've purchased—that make us into a corporation's billboard, with a company's logo or name emblazoned brightly across our chest. Sometimes it's deliberate; we're happy to advertise the local coffee house or our favorite band on a T-shirt because we identify with them. But sometimes our clothes are sending a message we don't want to be sending. We're promoting things we don't really want to support with our dollars and time because we've taken the path of least resistance and haven't bothered to get rid of the T-shirt. Today's the day to take back ownership of your brand.

Today — Go through your wardrobe (especially that T-shirt drawer) and get rid of anything you aren't comfortable and confident about advertising. Do you want to be a billboard for the local record store when you wear that Mary's Music T-shirt? How about the corporate store down the road? Your body is yours to control. You don't have to unwittingly be anyone's billboard.

— 123 —

Realize That You Want Memories, Not Regrets

I was a freshman in college and hopelessly enamored with a guy on campus. It was the most enamored I had ever been without being in a relationship, and the intensity of my feelings had me a bit undone. Scared of what I felt, scared of what could happen—either finding the love or heartbreak of my life—I was paralyzed. While this guy showed interest, I acted indifferent. I feigned interest in other people. I distracted myself because I was absolutely petrified that if he got to know me, he would no longer be interested. I was intimidated by the other women who showed interest in him. They seemed prettier, older, smarter, more sophisticated. They seemed like everything I was not and so I stalled.

On the last day of the semester, one of my best friends from high school picked me up and drove me home. In the car, I confessed my confusion about my crush—the other-worldliness of my emotions and feelings, my paralysis, my self-consciousness.

Erich's eyes darted away from the highway in front of us. He looked at me kindly and said, "If you keep acting the way you are acting, Rosie, you will only have regrets in your life. You will not have created any memories." It was a profound thing for a nineteen-year-old man to say. I sat with that truth the rest of the way home.

I later mustered up some courage in dealing with that crush, but it was never quite enough. Erich's words, however, were the kernel of insight I needed to readdress how I was approaching life in my new college setting. I was acting mostly out of fear and self-consciousness, when my youth had been marked by confidence and fearlessness. It reminded me to get back to myself, and to stay rooted in what I had to offer rather than in what I feared I lacked.

Today —— Imagine that Erich said those words to you. Consider what he said. Step away from dodging experiences, and step into making memories.

— 124 —

Find a Tailor

One of the best tips I've learned from a stylist friend is to find and use a great tailor. Not many clothes fit correctly right off the rack. A great seamstress or tailor can shorten sleeves, take in waists, reduce bulk, and do other sharp tailory things that will make your clothes suit you perfectly. And when your clothes fit you well, you feel better in them.

Today ⟶ Ask around for recommendations for a good tailor—don't wait until you have a need for one. Then go through your wardrobe to see if there is anything that could use some tweaking now. If so, visit the tailor to learn what he or she would do to improve the item's fit. If you feel good about the change and the person's skills, go for it.

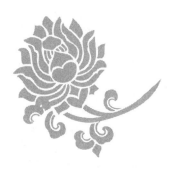

— 125 —

Understand that You Can Shape Your World

When I was doing the interviews for my book *Hijas Americanas*, I asked every woman if she'd ever had, or was considering, plastic surgery. One young woman startled me with her answer.

"Yes, I've had two nose jobs," she said. For a moment, I wondered if she had two noses (because how else could someone have had two nose jobs?). Then an image of Michael Jackson flashed in my mind. Got it.

She told me that when she was a teenager, her mom encouraged her to get a nose job. A major event in her life was approaching, and the mother worried that since her daughter had always hated her nose, she would hate the pictures from this event for the rest of her life. Trusting her mom's opinion, the girl met with a plastic surgeon, who said, "I see that we can do a few things to make you more comfortable with your nose. But your nose also shows your Indian ancestry, and I can't, in good conscience, do away with that. If you want to have the bridge of your nose altered, you'll need to see someone else." The young woman thought the doctor had a good plan that involved minimal changes to her nose, so she agreed to the surgery.

A few years later, she traveled to Colombia to visit family she had not seen in years. When they saw her, they were shocked to see that her nose looked similar to the way it always had.

"You live in America," they said. "Why would you have plastic surgery on your nose and still look like you are from Colombia?" They took her to a local plastic surgeon, who told her she needed an American nose (ever seen one of those?). In Colombia, she had her second nose-reshaping surgery.

Our interview occurred a few years after that trip. Reflecting on the surgeries, she told me, "I'm on my third nose, and what I know now is that my first nose was fine. I just wasn't sure enough of myself to know that back then, when people were suggesting that a nose job would make me happier."

That's just it, isn't it? We aren't always fully possessed enough to know that we can be in charge of our lives and bodies.

Today —— Understand that you can shape your world. You do not have to be shaped *by* your world. You can determine your own body and self-image. It does not have to be reflected back to you.

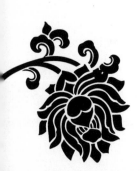

— 126 —

Get Over Size

E ver tried something on that you loved on the rack, only to find that you actually needed one size up? Did you try on a larger size, or did you think, *That's not my size,* and walk away from the cute piece of clothing? For too many women, size is a deal maker or breaker. We define ourselves by the number on the tag, and we only invest in clothes labeled with a number we are willing to swallow.

But the truth is, sizing is not universal. You can be a size 10 in one brand, an 8 in another, and a 12 in yet another brand. Size says nothing about you. It is more arbitrary than you realize. In fact, I am sometimes different sizes in the exact same brand, depending on how the designer cut the particular style.

Today —— Stop by a store and take three different sizes of a few different items you like into the dressing room. Don't look at the size when you try on the item, but see how each fits you. Choose which ones look and feel best. You don't have to purchase the items. Just go through the exercise of looking at fit rather than size.

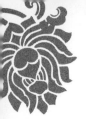

— 127 —

Be Kind

We all know the old adage "Beauty is as beauty does." It points out that it's personality, not physical attributes, that make a person beautiful, and it takes mean girls to task for how they act. It is likely that when you defined beauty in one of our earlier exercises, you at least included—perhaps even stressed—how a person acts in your definition.

Being kind to other people, recognizing and honoring the humanity that is all around you, does more than just warm the hearts of others. It also warms your heart by allowing you to bask in what you share, and it positively affects your sense of self.

Today — Be kind in every exchange you have. Watch how kindness encourages others and helps you to feel your best too.

—•• 128 ••—

Don't Take Things Personally

T oo often, our view of the world is myopic. The unkind sales clerk at the drugstore must not find us attractive; the terse quip from our coworker shows that he doesn't think we're funny; the darting eyes of the person we're approaching means he can't stand the sight of us. Oh, how we can make things all about us, eroding our confidence, when the situation is likely not about us at all.

Today ⟶ Think about all the messages you could have inadvertently sent to someone else when you were lost in thought, mulling over some sad news, or not feeling well. Now, think about how many times you may have interpreted someone else's distracted moments as messages to you. Very rarely is someone else's mood or reaction—especially when that someone is a person you don't know very well—about you. Before you allow yourself to spiral into sadness over the perceived diss, remind yourself that it is likely not personal.

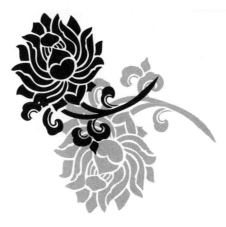

DAY

—— 129 ——

Remember That Scars Show Character

I n my early twenties, I fell down my apartment stairs. I was on the way to pick up my friend Ben at the time; Ben and I still engage in a spirited debate over what caused the fall and who was responsible for the resulting scar.

The short of it is that my knee split open, leaving a three-inch wide wound, and I never went to the hospital to have it stitched up. Ultimately, the wound closed, leaving an inch-long scar. It is jagged, like the silhouette of a mountain range, and it serves as a reminder of that wretched fall.

I once dated a man who looked at that scar, traced its outline, and said "Scars show character." While he was referring to my physical landscape, I couldn't help but interpret it as also describing my emotional landscape. He won me over in that moment, affirming what I had always believed: It is the difficult things that make your life rich. Tough times give your life personality and flavor in a way that easy times cannot.

Today —— Remember that our scars, both the physical and the emotional, show character. When I see the marks from chicken pox on my upper lip, I remember the sixteen-year-old girl who battled that virus. She traveled to Seattle, Washington, for a conference after she was no longer contagious but still covered in the scabs of illness. The desire to see the Pacific Northwest was so on fire within her that she wouldn't cancel the trip.

When I feel the heat of anxiety lick at my neck just as I board an airplane, I recall that I come by my fear of flying honestly, after losing two of the people I loved most in a plane crash in the 1990s. I am grateful, in that moment, for my capacity to love unconditionally, even if someone is not my blood relative and even if it means I might lose them.

Think of your own emotional and physical scars and reframe your experiences with them so that you can see the depth of your character that they reveal.

— 130 —

Celebrate Something

Many of us, especially when we struggle with confidence, tend to undervalue moments in our lives. We get a performance-based raise at work and don't want to mention it to friends because we don't want to make them feel bad or to seem like we're bragging. We make inroads on a long-term goal and just swallow the news because we don't want to jinx it. We minimize things so much that we begin to believe they don't matter, but they do.

Today —— Celebrate something for yourself that you normally wouldn't. Maybe you call together a group of friends to go out for a toast or call a family member so that you can share your good news. Take a moment to really appreciate what normally wouldn't warrant your appreciation.

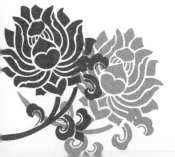

— 131 —

Commit to Buying Only What Fits

We've all been there, eyeing something we love at the store, then buying it regardless of how it will look on our bodies. What do we end up with? Not a lovely wardrobe that is perfectly our style but a bunch of things that just tease us with their too-small shape or drape and cover us because they are too big. By buying things that do not fit, we negate our bodies and ourselves. We might be saying that it doesn't matter whether or not our bodies are comfortable or presentable. We could be saying that our bodies are the only things people need to consider in understanding us. We could be saying we hate our bodies or don't respect our bodies. None of those are statements we should be making.

Today —— From this day forward, commit to buying only things that fit you. Not sure what a good fit looks like? Shop with a discerning friend who seems to wear her clothes well (not someone whose clothes wear her) and get her input.

— 132 —

Hug

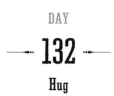

After seeing my parents, my husband always mentions how much he loves my mom's hugs. She's a good hugger, the kind of person who holds you close and just wraps you in her little arms. Truth be told, my husband doesn't just enjoy the hug itself. He also enjoys the benefits that come from that hug. Hugging usually leaves us feeling less stressed; it creates a sense of calm and builds a sense of connection. That sense of well-being is just the thing to boost one's confidence and esteem.

Today ⟶ Hug the people closest to you in your life and let each hug linger just a bit. With each embrace, you are enhancing your relationship and your sense of self. You are also boosting the other person's self-esteem, letting them know how loveable they really are.

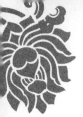

Remember That We Are All Susan Boyle

If you own a television or a computer, you caught wind of the Susan Boyle story in 2009. A forty-seven-year-old Scottish lady gets the chance to sing for her life on *Britain's Got Talent,* and it turns out, she's got quite the voice.

My favorite Broadway play is *Les Miserables,* so I was excited to see Susan Boyle sing *I Dreamed a Dream.* What I wasn't prepared for was how the audience reacted to her initially. I almost had to turn the video clip off before she started singing because watching the way Ms. Boyle was judged initially, before she shared her talent, unsettled me. The clip went viral and millions watched, cheering Ms. Boyle all the way.

Like many other people, I found the media hoopla surrounding her a bit condescending. It felt like, "You didn't look like we thought you should, and sound like we thought you should, so let's dwell on how unbelievable it is that *you* can sing like that." But I did get why everyday people—me and maybe you—went to YouTube over and over again to see the video. We've all felt like Susan Boyle at some time or another, and watching her performance is like finally seeing the bully get taken down.

"While I watched the clip, I couldn't help but think about the particular song she was singing," my friend Jill said. "The words made me cry: *But the tigers come at night with their voices soft as thunder, as they tear your hope apart and they turn your dream to shame.* I kept thinking about how this didn't feel like a random song, but it was her song to this audience and the media."

While I was never really curious about Boyle's life back in the village and how she felt about the reaction she received (I just wanted to hear her sing again), I was curious about the people in that audience—the ones who had such a negative reaction to Ms. Boyle when she walked onto the stage and said she wanted her chance. How has their thinking changed since seeing what they saw in person, hearing what they heard, and knowing the sounds and faces and judgments they made in that auditorium? Are they less quick to judge now? Are they more willing to give people the benefit of the doubt? Do they offer grace more often? It's not enough for us to get to a place in the world where we are willing to cheer on the underdog once they've impressed us, willing to have exceptions to the rule once they prove their worthiness to be an exception. Wouldn't it be great if we didn't assign value to someone—underdog or top-dog value—based on appearance? Let's hold our arms wide open for anyone's possibility, a place where there are no rules based on universal standards of beauty.

Today —— Consider this: Susan Boyle's confidence, her passion, her good humor, her pluck, and her immeasurable joy in singing were really contagious. Beauty, as we viscerally know—which is why millions of us have connected with this video—does not fit into just one box. It's bigger, more dramatic, more marvelous, more encompassing than that, and all of us, inherently, have it. What moments have taught you this in your life? How can you hold onto them as shining examples of how you want to approach the world?

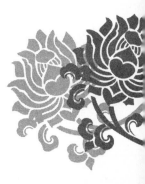

— 134 —

Practice One In, One Out

Ff I'm not disciplined about it, I can be the queen of holding on to things that don't suit me, don't fit, aren't my style, or don't reflect who I am anymore. So almost a decade ago, after a day spent cleaning my closet, I came up with a new rule for myself. From that day forward, I adopted a "One In, One Out" policy. If I purchase something new for my wardrobe—shoes, slacks, a jean jacket, or whatever—I have to donate at least one item from my wardrobe. I don't have to swap shoes for shoes, but I do have to acknowledge that my good fortune should be shared. The practice also helps me be more deliberate about keeping a wardrobe that reflects who I am at the moment, not who I was ten years ago or will be fifteen pounds from now.

Today —— Think about the items you have purchased for your wardrobe in the last month and count 'em up. Yes, even count the $9.99 T-shirts from Target. Then, head to your closet and do a purge, pulling out at least that many items to be donated to a local charity or clothing closet. Practice the One In, One Out rule next time you make a purchase.

Need some help finding a place to donate your clothes? Look for a local chapter of Dress for Success or call your local United Way or YMCA for ideas.

Write Yourself a Note

S ometimes a motivating reminder at just the right time—or when you least expect it—can be the buoy that keeps us afloat.

Today ➤—➤ Write yourself several short, inspiring notes that mean something to you. Next, drop those notes in a few places where you'll find them later—a gym bag, purse, sunglass case, make-up drawer, or wherever. You might even type yourself a positive message as an appointment in your computer calendar, so that you'll be surprised with it days or weeks from now. By putting inspirational notes out there for future discovery, you are setting yourself up for a future bout of positivity that just might arrive when you need it most.

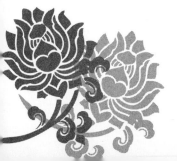

— 136 —

Don't Be Afraid to Ask "Why Do You Ask?"

O ne of the topics we discuss each semester in my body image seminar is how race, class, culture, and religion impact body image. As you might imagine, it is infinitely interesting to discuss these topics. Often, the notion of a "box of understanding" comes up in the conversation.

Perhaps it's human nature to want to put people or things into boxes so we can understand them better. "If I know X about you, then I can assume Y is true for you," we say, and then we decipher people by these categories rather than patiently and generously giving them room for their unique wholeness.

One of my students told us how disappointed someone was when she responded to his question "What are you?" with the answer "Black."

"Oh," he told her. "I thought you might have Filipino in you." Suddenly, he was treating her like she was a lot less interesting.

We talked about what she could have said to her friend, or what anyone might say in a situation when she's dealing with someone who is operating within a very narrowing box of understanding. We wanted an option that would allow a graceful response, even if she suspects the inquisitor is rude, racist, classist, or otherwise mean.

My suggestion: Always answer an inappropriate or awkward question with a question.

Are you mixed? Where are you from? What are your parents? What are you?

The perfect response: Why do you ask?

Today ⟶ Don't be afraid to ask "Why do you ask?" when faced with an inappropriate question. "Why do you ask?" gives the person an opportunity to rethink his or her approach, to consider why he or she needs or wants to ask this question. It also reminds them that you are a real person who might possibly be hurt or offended by the question; it reintroduces the parameters of polite conversation. Finally, it gives you the chance to gauge the sincerity of the question and to decide how you wish to answer it. It is not your responsibility to answer everything that is asked of you. You have the right to share only information you feel comfortable with—to maintain boundaries and to keep yourself safe.

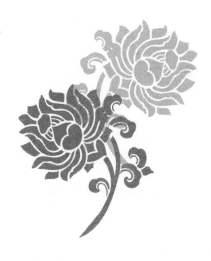

— 137 —

Consider Careers

Sometimes I ask people in my journaling workshops to list some careers they would just love—for whatever reason—even if they don't have the skills to do them. If I had to write my own list today, it would look like this: foundation officer, creativity consultant, professional organizer, torch singer, radio personality, private investigator, television sports announcer, and professional athlete.

I have people create this list because I want them to think about what interests and intrigues them about these dream careers. Once they know, they can consider incorporating those things into their everyday lives.

For example, I'd love to be a professional athlete not because I like competing, want to be famous, or want to make a lot of money, but because I love to be in motion and to stretch my body's capabilities. What can I do with that information if I am being true to myself? I can dedicate some time each week to athletic pursuits that I enjoy and that stretch me (literally and figuratively).

Am I really going to go out and earn my credentials to be a private investigator? Probably not—but it does explain my fascination with reading memoir, watching *Dateline* and *20/20,* conducting research for my work, and asking too many questions of most everyone I meet. I continue to do those things because they feed my well. And feeding my well is another way of saying that I am catering to my soul, which is an essential part of enhancing my sense of well-being.

What does any of this have to do with self-image and body image? So often we do things out of habit and expectation, not because they interest us or ignite our passion. When we live a life that is accidental, one that is not in touch with who we are at the core, we begin to lose ourselves and our way. When we lose ourselves and our way, we lose our confidence. And when we lose our confidence, our body image and self-image can go all to hell.

Today ⟿ In your *Beautiful You* journal, list ten careers you would love to have—the skills, training, and lifestyle you have right now notwithstanding. Now look over your list and consider what it can teach you about yourself. Are you living in a way that plugs into what this list tells you? If so, how? If not, what's the first step you can take to start doing so?

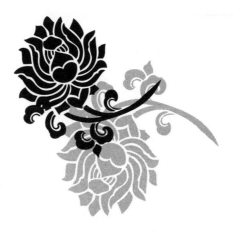

— 138 —

Consider the Unresolved Issue in Your Life

While journaling provides you with a way to vent your emotions, it also helps you see which issues have taken too much of your priceless energy. Vent about something often enough and you will realize that it is taking away valuable time from something else. Journaling can serve as a tool to write *through* something as opposed to about something. It can also serve as a call to resolve issues.

Today —— In your *Beautiful You* journal, reflect on these questions. What issue consumes the greatest amount of your brainpower and emotional energy? Perhaps it is your weight, your romantic relationship, your professional life, your familial relationship, or your finances. Whatever it is, consider for a moment what your life would be like if this issue were resolved. Write about that in your *Beautiful You* journal. What would you gain from having the issue resolved? How would you spend your extra time and energy? Understand that every day you put off deciding on whether or how to resolve this issue, you are actually making the choice to keep the issue alive in your life. If that's what you're doing, what lessons do you still need to learn to realize your best self? What are the possibilities for you? Consider what steps are worth taking now (and what steps you are ready to take) and move forward with them, toward growth.

— 139 —

Consider Your Role Models

Thinking about our role models helps us consider our values, desires, and visions. Living a life that is centered on those three things leads to a greater sense of satisfaction.

Today —— Answer these questions in your *Beautiful You* journal: Who are your role models? Why are they your role models? What do you have in common with them?

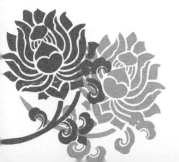

— 140 —

Harness Your Jealousy

Jealousy. It's insidious. Not for the object of your jealous feelings. No, it's insidious for you when you feel it—it's like a cancer growing in your body. Eventually, jealousy makes you dissatisfied with everything. You become more uncomfortable psychologically with every flash of green.

Today ⟶ Use your jealousy as a motivator for action. In your *Beautiful You* journal, consider what makes you feel jealous. What positive goal can you set for yourself that uses that emotion to help you accomplish or change something? Make that goal and go for it.

— 141 —

Make Nervousness Good Energy

Sometimes our nerves completely undo us. But it is possible to turn nervousness into good, positive energy.

Today — Think about something you have coming up that might make you nervous. Maybe it's an exam, a paper, a presentation, an interview. Whatever it is, go ahead and channel that anxiety into a useful feeling by thoroughly preparing for the upcoming event. Realize that your anxiety is simply telling you that the event matters to you. If it matters to you, you should devote extra time to making sure you can do your best. Give yourself plenty of opportunity to prepare. When the event approaches and you feel anxious, realize that your subconscious is telling you that you care, that you are hoping for the best possible outcome in this situation, and that you should go for it.

DAY

— 142 —

Face Your Fears

When I am home alone at night, I find it difficult to sleep. I have an active imagination and I can easily finish the story of what happens to the woman who is home alone on a dark, dreary, winter night. In fact, I can write that story 100 different ways, all of them equally terrifying. So I stay up. The television fills my bedroom with noise, as if sound can distract me from what I fear.

Worry. It can eat at us. One of my friends calls her worry habit "catastrophizing." She makes a catastrophe out of her life and then just keeps it going in her head until she is paralyzed and cannot take action. Worrying paralyzes us, keeps us from becoming our best selves. It splinters our confidence, distorts our self-awareness, and steals our future right out from under us.

Today —— Face your fears. Open up your *Beautiful You* journal and write down every worry that pops into your mind. If you wish, divide your worries into two categories—Professional/Educational/Vocational and Personal. Next, review the list and decide what you can do about each worry. Write down one actionable step—an action you can take right now toward alleviating that worry—next to each item. Copy those actionable steps onto your regular to-do list. Can't think of an actionable step for one of your items? Then let that worry go. You can't allow yourself to be consumed by something that your energy and effort cannot control. Picture that item written on a helium balloon, and then picture yourself letting that balloon loose into the universe. Watch the balloon float far, far away; that worry is dissipating in your mind's eye. If it comes back to you later (and worry is sneaky like that) envision the balloon again being set free into the universe.

— 143 —

Breathe

Somewhere along the way, we learned that if you are mad or need to collect yourself, you should stop and take ten deep breaths. While it might seem the trick worked because it separated you for a moment from the event that had upset you, it turns out that slow, deep breathing actually helps dissipate stress, leading to a calmer, happier you.

Today —— Close your eyes. Think of a tranquil setting that brings you peace. Now take ten deep breaths that fill up your chest. Exhale each breath with an audible sigh and visualize any negative feelings, tensions, and stress leaving your body with each breath.

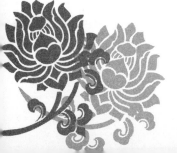

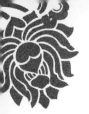

— 144 —

Examine Your Reactions

O ften when we interact with people who are difficult, we later reflect on what their behaviors and choices did to us. That reflection can be valuable. It can show us what our boundaries are, what gives us anxiety, what we need in our relationships. But we don't always go to that place—the place that gives us insight about ourselves—when we reflect. Sometimes we just harp on the other person, not giving ourselves the opportunity to grow.

Today —— In your *Beautiful You* journal, consider what your reactions to other people say about you. Does your anxiety around a coworker illuminate what makes you feel insecure? Does your anger at your partner indicate your boundaries? Does your frustration with a friend reflect what you need in relationships? Today, consider each reaction you have to a person in your life and what perspective you can gain by examining it. By learning from our cues, we obtain self understanding, an essential trait on our quest to greater confidence.

— 145 —

Stop Apologizing

A woman I adore is a chronic apologizer. It is honorable to take respon-sibility for the things we do, but her apologies are never necessary. Her apologies, sadly, are more a measure of how she feels about herself. She's not nearly as confident as she should be, and her apologies—her fear that she is always doing something wrong—announce that insecurity. When you apologize constantly, for things you haven't really done wrong, you are diminishing yourself, your presence, and your ideas.

Today ——⟶ Stop apologizing for things that do not really need your apol-ogy (calling someone and apologizing for interrupting her day). And while you're at it, quit diminishing yourself and your ideas ("This is probably a dumb idea."). If you want to offer someone the opportunity to tell you it's not a great time to talk, simply ask, "Is right now an okay time?" If you want to communicate that you are not wedded to your suggestion, say, "I'm not hooked on this, but one option might be…" and then complete the sen-tence. By changing the language you use to talk about yourself, you begin to acknowledge your own worth.

— 146 —

Finish This Sentence

Sometimes we just need a reminder of our beauty and brilliance.

Today —— In your *Beautiful You* journal, finish this sentence:

I feel beautiful when . . .

Now reflect upon the answer. When was the last time you allowed yourself to do what makes you feel beautiful?

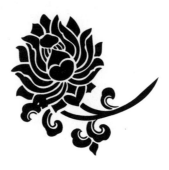

— 147 —

Make Over Your 'Do

I wouldn't think a haircut could make that big of a difference if I hadn't experienced good and bad haircuts myself. A stylist who knows just the right haircut for your hair and face can make such a difference in how you feel about your hair, and thus, yourself. In fact, in a study by the hair-care company Pantene, at least 75 percent of women reported that a "bad hair day" affects their self-confidence. With the right haircut, you can avoid that dip in your confidence.

Today —— Look through magazines and online to find photos of haircuts you like, and if you don't already have a stylist you love, ask around for recommendations. Make an appointment and go in ready to hear what the stylist thinks will work for you; now give it a whirl. If what he or she suggests is a change too drastic for you to feel comfortable with at once, work with the stylist on a plan that can get you there over a couple appointments.

— 148 —

Examine What Healthy Means to You

D o you spend a significant amount of time working out in the gym or outdoors, chasing an image of "healthy" that is dangling before you like a carrot? Is that image your own or did it come from someone else? While we can all agree that good health is important, "healthy" is not a one-size-fits-all concept. Unless our standards and behaviors take our particular realities into account, it will be impossible for us to realize a healthy life for ourselves.

Today —— Answer these questions in your *Beautiful You* journal. What does being healthy mean to you? What does it look like? What does it feel like? What will or does it take for you to achieve good health?

— 149 —

Greet People

As a girl and young adult, I said hello to everyone I passed in the school hallway or in the mall. Even when I drove past someone, I always waved my fingers in a greeting.

"Why do you wave to everyone?" my first love once asked me as we were driving down the road.

"I just think it's nice to acknowledge people," I answered.

In my mid-twenties, I traveled to Germany to visit a dear friend who was stationed there as an Army First Lieutenant. Germany was my birthplace, and it was my first trip back since my family left the country when I was two. I practiced my Guten Tags and other German phrases in anticipation of rediscovering my birth country.

And then I realized that Germany is not the type of place where you randomly greet strangers. In fact, it is the type of place where someone will tell you that you are being too loud if you laugh boisterously in a restaurant. Don't try it, I already did.

So a week into my German adventure, and a little brokenhearted that the country didn't love me nearly as much as I loved its lush vegetation, surprising little castles, grand cathedrals, roadside flower vendors, red phone booths, and Mini Coopers, I decided to take matters into my own hands. I decided to greet people even if they weren't willing to greet me back.

At a beer festival in Wiesbaden, a city I adore, I walked the streets saying Guten Tag to every person I passed. I smiled. I made eye contact. I watched as people giggled in sheer surprise at the greeting. Sometimes people even stopped for a moment, perplexed, as if they were thinking, "What do I do with that greeting?" Two hours in, a man about my age said hello back and kept walking. It felt like victory.

It's so easy to get caught up in the intricacies of our lives, to lose sight of the road in front of us and, perhaps worse, to lose sight of the people right in front of us. When we do that, we aren't celebrating or even living in the moment. Our minds are focused somewhere else—the future, the past, anywhere but the now. But we exist, all of us, in the now. By being as present, as real, as accessible in the now as we can possibly be, we show up and we engage the world with the best version of ourselves. And bringing out that self is championing our brilliance.

Today —— Greet people as you pass them in the hallway at school, the corridor at work, the parking lot, the grocery store, or on the road while you're driving. Let them know that it was worth it for you to take a moment to acknowledge them, and let yourself know that it is worth it for you to be present in each moment.

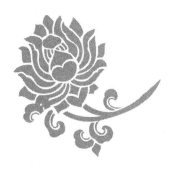

— 150 —

Affirm Your Body

Our bodies allow us to experience so much, and yet we spend more time belittling them for what we perceive they are lacking or do not give us than we do affirming them.

Today — Be satisfied with your body in its role as your vehicle for experiencing life. Take a moment to thank your body for allowing you that experience.

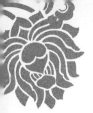

— 151 —

Write a Gratitude List for Your Day

Too often, we fail to see the miracles and beauty in our days. Yet gratitude is such an important contributor to our sense of happiness and well-being. The Gratitude Journal gained fame after Oprah Winfrey featured it on her show. The concept, which comes from the Quaker tradition, is to write a gratitude list that celebrates three to five things, no matter how small, each night. By grounding yourself in the things for which you are grateful, you become even more empowered to explore your life's possibilities.

Today — Open up your *Beautiful You* Journal and write down five things you were especially grateful for in your day.

— 152 —

Infuse Your Space with Meaning

"This is so clearly your classroom," my friend Jen said when she visited me at school one day.

As I looked around, I could see that she was right. My classroom brimmed with my spirit: bright posters bearing inspirational quotes and lots of personal mementos on my desk—a piece of sea glass worn into a brilliant blue, a tiny box with a tinier painting inside that a friend gave me after a difficult moment in college. The space that I inhabited for countless hours each week was comfortable to me because I had taken the time to infuse it with the flavors of my life. Everywhere I looked in that space, I could see keepsakes that were linked to a particular memory, friendship, value, or goal. Because that space inspired me, it helped me try to inspire my students every day.

Today —— Think about the places where you spend the most time and think about the personal tokens you display in each location. These are the mementos that help you feel grounded, connected, and inspired when you see them. If you don't have anything of personal meaning on display, take the time to make these spaces more inspirational.

— 153 —

Embrace What You Avoid

Do you avoid eye contact with yourself in the mirror because you don't like your face? Do you ignore your feet because you can't stand the sight of them? By avoiding a part of our bodies, we are, in essence, avoiding ourselves. It is impossible to nurture our whole selves if we don't embrace our entirety.

Today —— If you regularly avoid looking at or caring for a part of your body, choose to embrace it for today. If you don't love your feet, go for a pedicure or sit down and patiently massage them with a moisturizing cream. If you look away from the mirror every time you wash your hands, try gazing at your face without judgment. By turning off the negative racket in your head and learning that you can be nonjudgmental about yourself, you begin to see and celebrate your whole person.

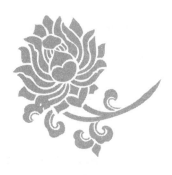

— 154 —

Buy Yourself Flowers

During my first year as a college administrator, I participated in a student service trip to Brazil. An English professor and I were leading the trip, and we often got together to plan the details of our journey. Our frequent meetings usually took place in her office, a comfortable space that reflected her distinct style. I noticed that she always had a beautiful vase of fresh flowers on display. Annie was married to another English professor, and I figured that Randy, her dear husband, was behind those flowers.

One day, just as I was about to leave, I looked over at her bright tulips, my favorite flowers, and said, "I love that you always have fresh flowers."

Her response: "I buy them for myself every week."

Buying yourself flowers? Such a simple act of self-love and such an easy way to bring beauty into your life.

A few years later, with the idea to start my own weekly flowers tradition, I bought a beautiful robin's-egg-blue vase that was made and glazed by a North Carolina potter. Every Saturday from April to October, I amble down to our local farmer's market and spend a few minutes looking through the various bouquets offered for sale. The blooms are always enormous and inexpensive. I always find flowers I have never seen before, and when I hand over $10 for my Miss-America-size bouquet, I know that I am caring for and honoring myself.

Today — Stop at a floral shop, a farmers market, or even on the side of the road. Buy (or pick) yourself some flowers to enjoy for the coming week.

— 155 —

Let Go of That Girl

Somewhere in your head is the woman you thought you should, would, could, or had to be. The thing about her is, she likely isn't who you were meant to become. Instead, she is a compilation of other things—messages you received, looks you envied, things you thought mattered. She isn't you. She's taunting you. And it's time to let her go.

Today —— Who was the person you've always thought you had to be? In your *Beautiful You* journal, capture her essence, down to her lipstick shade and way of life. Then say goodbye to her, letting her know why she doesn't make sense for the woman that you have become. It is only when we release ourselves from these false attachments to an idea of us that we actually give ourselves room to become our best, most authentic selves.

— 156 —

Sit Outside for Five

Our baby boy was so sad to say goodbye to his caregiver in Ethiopia when we traveled there to finalize the adoption and bring him back to the United States. His woeful cry that first day seemed endless. We were ready to try anything, but fortunately we discovered early on that nothing soothed him like time outside, where he could see trees and wildlife and breathe the fresh air. Even today, almost two years later, being outside continues to be our salve, our go-to remedy for tears or anxiety. As it turns out, it is not just soothing to our boy. Being outside is good medicine for us, too.

Jolina Ruckert, a researcher at the University of Washington, says, "Many neglect to realize how connections to the natural world are necessary for humans to flourish. There's a lot of research suggesting that experiencing nature is therapeutic. Being in nature helps us recuperate, relax, and reflect, among a myriad of other physiological and psychological benefits."

She continues: "We need nature. For much of our evolutionary history, we have had deep, complex relationships with the natural world. A need to interact with nature is deeply ingrained in the architecture of our minds. Our relationship with nature is part of who we are and what it means to be human."

Today —— Step outside, find a peaceful spot, and just enjoy it—no matter the weather—for five minutes. Observing nature reminds us of the visual variety and sheer beauty that exists all around us: a hydrangea bush is shocking in its colors, an oak tree is majestic in its stance, each red cardinal that flashes by you is equally radiant. The appreciation we have for nature is the appreciation we should have for the beauty and variety of human life. Stepping outside helps remind us of that truth; it also helps center us.

DAY

157

Forgive Others

Here is what I have learned over the years about those who inflict pain on other people. It's rarely, if ever, about us. It's almost always about that person and what is missing in his or her life. The person who has said or done awful things to me? Her actions really aren't a reflection of me. Those actions are a reflection of what she is missing or mourning or considering or ignoring in her own life. If I hold onto her words and actions—if I add them up, as if they somehow have meaning—I'm working off a false premise that keeps me from protecting and honoring myself. If I allow myself to harbor resentments toward the person that wasn't kind to me, I am really only limiting my own life.

Today — Consider the people in your life whose words or actions have hurt you or your understanding of yourself. Think about how their actions may have actually been a reflection of their own lives, not yours. In your *Beautiful You* journal, write each of these people a letter (you don't have to mail it) and offer them a quiet forgiveness. Then move forward, choosing to embrace the peace in your heart.

— 158 —

Forgive Yourself

Sometimes the person you most need to forgive is yourself. We often say terrible things to ourselves, put ourselves in unspeakable situations. We wage war on ourselves, call ourselves names, limit our own abilities— even though we would never do these things to anyone else. We live by a double standard when we treat ourselves as second-class citizens. We can learn to give ourselves the same kindnesses we so willingly give to others.

Polly Campbell suffers from juvenile rheumatoid arthritis. She has always offered others grace and forgiveness but found it hard to do the same for herself.

"I used to think, 'I am not pretty enough. I am not thin enough. I cannot walk the same way other people do.' Finally, I just looked at myself a different way and said, 'Thank you, body. I am living my life thanks to you.' When I shifted from a place of 'I am not enough' to a place of gratitude, I learned a lot about forgiveness. I am working as hard as I can. I am living the best life I can. When I stepped out of a place in which I was not enough, I stepped into this place of forgiveness."

Today — Forgive yourself for the berating you have done or the power you have given away. Offer yourself kind words of forgiveness, and understand that the power of this forgiveness may not be felt immediately. You may need to reissue those words of apology for several days before the relief settles in.

DAY

159

Dance

In high school, I had the good fortune of going to a weeklong leader-ship camp each summer. In many ways I was vibrant: I was unafraid, a conduit of energy and warmth. But this camp started each morning with something called the "Energizer." It was a 20-minute dance party, and it was the bane of my existence. While hundreds of kids got up and shook it, I sat in a chair and watched. I was there because I had held leadership positions, experiences that should indicate I had confidence, and yet I was always too self-conscious to let myself go and dance. When I started college, I quickly realized that the weekend social scene was anchored by dance parties and drinking. I didn't drink and so that left me with one other option—dancing. What I learned quickly was that most people were too consumed in their own dancing (or drinking) to really care about how I looked. I started to dance and loved it. I invented my own line dance. I found a dance partner who would toss me every which way, even upside down, always bringing me gently back to my feet. I couldn't get enough of it. At my sister's bachelor-ette party, I danced into the wee hours of the morning, buoyed by one of her bridesmaids who looked at me and said, "You are such a fun dancer." My fear of not being able to dance well kept me from doing it for so long and made me so self-conscious. It is ironic that in the end I embraced dancing and it has made me more confident.

Today —— Turn up the music and dance. You can do it in the privacy of your own home with no one watching or go out to a club. The point is sim-ply to move and enjoy the release your body feels as you let go.

Don't Force a Storyline

On our journey home from Ethiopia, we traveled through Dubai. There, a lovely female airline employee stopped us, taken by our boy and struck, I am sure, by the fact that he didn't look like either of us. We talked a bit about the adoption, about being parents, about Ethiopia, and then we turned to make our way to the ticket counter.

"Don't worry," she called out to us. "Now you'll get pregnant. I just know it."

People are inspired to adopt for many different reasons, and only sometimes do those reasons have to do with infertility. Infertility, in fact, had nothing to do with our decision. Adoption was our first choice and the only way we envisioned building our family. When our little guy came to us so serendipitously, we saw even more clearly that our family was coming together just the way it was intended to come together.

"Did she just say what I think she said?" my husband asked after the sweet airline employee had shouted her reassurances after us.

"Yeah," I said, shrugging if off and shifting the baby to my other hip.

"Oh, wow," he said, and he shook his head.

But what she said had nothing on what someone said to me at my nephew's baptism a few years before we adopted our son. There I was, holding my nephew and minding my own business, when my sister's sister-in-law asked if she could hold the baby.

"Absolutely," I said and handed the little guy to her.

"Oh, don't take that baby from Rosie," a woman interjected. "She clearly needs to hold onto him a little longer so that the baby bug will bite her."

I walked into the kitchen and cleaned the meatball dish because it was better than standing around and making conversation with someone who would say that to a woman she's only met once and whom she knew nothing about.

It's a funny thing we do to each other—especially to girls and young women. We force a certain storyline on them. We call our girls princesses and have them dress up as brides at the youngest of ages. But the princess rarely saves herself in the story, and the bride is always waiting for her groom. We don't ask or force boys to play in the same way. When a girl comes home from kindergarten, we ask her if she has a boyfriend—not whether or not she's kicking the ball far at recess or if she's doing great with her numbers or letters. We don't ask the girlfriend question to a little boy with the same regularity, vigor, teasing, or expectation. When a high school girl has a boyfriend, we wonder—often aloud—if that's her husband to be. Again, we don't do the same thing with our boys. When a young woman is dating a young man, we ask if he's the one; might they get engaged; when? Most young men are given room around that question. Once a couple is married, people begin questioning the wife fairly frequently about kids. And once the first baby comes, when are you going to start working on number two?

I asked my husband sometime before our family plans were concrete if he was ever asked about having a family.

"Never," he answered. "Why would someone ask?"

"That's a pretty personal question," he continued. "I mean, what if we couldn't get pregnant or something. Isn't the person who asks just asking for it?"

Why yes, honey, they are. And yet, it didn't keep people I hardly knew from frequently asking me and then trying to rationalize their inappropriate questions by adding, "I just ask because you both would be such great parents."

In the body image seminar I teach, we always talk about the storylines we give our boys and girls and how those storylines affect their self-image, body image, and choices. What I want more than anything in the world for our young people (and us adults) is the gift of room—the opportunity to make the choices and decisions they want and need to make without the weight of the world's expectations on them.

As a parent, I hope to be even more cognizant of it. I want our boy—and any other children we may one day have or adopt—to have the room to do what he wants, any time he wants it. I want him to not worry about being a writer because his mom writes or being a rugby player because his daddy was. I want him to own who he is every day without worrying about what the world expects from him. I want him, every day, to just proudly, meaningfully, playfully *be*. If we give that to our children, what we are really doing is placing the world, and all of its wonder, gently in the palms of their hands.

Today —— Watch your words and questions before you speak. Are you imposing a preconceived storyline onto your child, friend, or partner? Can you keep yourself from saying those words and allow that person to develop her story just as she wishes?

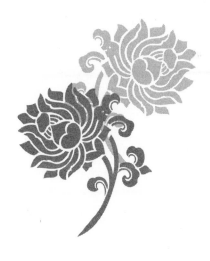

— 161 —

Wear Sunscreen

"Ladies and Gentlemen of the class of '99, wear sunscreen. If I could offer you only one tip for the future, sunscreen would be it."

So begins the popular ditty "Everybody's Free" (to wear sunscreen) released in the late 1990s by Baz Luhrmann. Luhrmann may have turned those words into song, but it was Mary Schmich of the *Chicago Tribune,* who actually wrote those words in her June 1, 1997, column titled "Advice, Like Youth, Probably Just Wasted on the Young."

All that said, what matters right now are those two words near the beginning of this page. Wear sunscreen. Taking care of your skin is a symbol that you are taking care of yourself and, most important, it protects you from skin cancer.

Today —— Apply a broad-spectrum sunscreen (you want one that protects against UVA and UVB rays) on all of your exposed skin.

— 162 —

Be a Body Warrior

One of the regular features on my blog immediately after the release of *Hijas Americanas* was "A Body Warrior to Meet." Each week I featured a woman of any age, shape, size, culture, race, religion, or background who was reclaiming herself—and redefining standards—by embracing her own unique beauty. It's not that these women don't have days when their self-esteem wavers, but they *are* living deliberately, with the intention of outwitting, out-charming, and outsmarting all that "you're not good enough!" chatter.

Today —— You too can become a Body Warrior. Open up your *Beautiful You* journal and complete the statements below, which I posed to the women I featured on my blog. (Want to be featured there yourself? Visit www.rosiemolinary.com.)

What I love about myself:

My biggest challenge in accepting my body and beauty:

My biggest support in learning to appreciate myself:

Beauty is:

Why I am strong:

Why I am beautiful:

What women must know:

— 163 —

Change the Default Setting of Your Mind

We've been working on positive thinking for a while now. Do you find that your mind is still centered on finding fault or are you able to keep it neutral? Today we are reemphasizing the importance of changing your way of thinking, a key step in moving toward satisfaction and positivity.

Today — Every time your mind turns to thoughts about yourself today, make sure that your thinking reflects a sense of satisfaction with yourself, your body, your looks. If you are looking in a mirror at the gym and aren't happy with what you find yourself thinking, command your mind to focus on your strength. If you are engaging with someone you haven't seen for awhile and find yourself wondering what she thinks of you, think about what a gift you can give her by paying attention to what she is really saying. As you begin to switch your way of thinking to one that emphasizes satisfaction, you'll notice that the ability to take pleasure and feel good starts to run deeper.

— 164 —

Concentrate on Touch

Perhaps the single most overwhelming experience of my life occurred the day a nanny handed me my baby boy in Addis Ababa, Ethiopia. He was solid; his weight represented the love the nannies at his care house had given him during his five-month stay. His hair was soft, the edges gently curling and hinting at the tight ringlets that would come later. His breath smelled of formula, a milky scent that I would come to love over the next few months. When he realized his nanny was leaving, and that he was being left with me and my husband—his new father—his cry cut to my soul. It signaled the shattering of a heart that we would have to put back together for him with our bottomless love.

I carried him in my arms as he cried, strolling back and forth in the courtyard of our guesthouse then pacing the living room. I rubbed his back and sang him soft choruses from "The Rose," by Bette Midler, the song that popped into my head at the moment, even though I hadn't heard it since eighth grade. Later, I would come to understand that the message from "The Rose" may have been the most appropriate one for the occasion.

Soon, our baby fell asleep in my arms, his head heavy on my shoulder, his breathing ragged from an upper respiratory infection, a tear still dotting his eye. I rubbed his back, breathed him in, felt his weight against me. And suddenly the enormity of it all was too much. We were sitting down, and I looked at my husband and calmly said, "I need you to take the baby. I am going to faint." He did, and I did.

I am often too careful or too busy, not as fully sensory as I should be or can be. In the days leading up to our adoption, I was efficient, checking things off, getting things done, preparing. But preparing a home isn't the same as preparing one's heart and mind.

That day in Addis Ababa, I experienced everything there was to experience about having a new son. To fully prepare both my heart and mind, I had to feel the hugeness, the vastness, the intensity of it. I felt it so acutely, all at once, that I needed to check out for a second to catch up with it.

I am grateful that my senses were so alive that day. Now I have every single detail about that experience ready so I can tell my son about it as he grows up.

Today —— Concentrate on touch. When you dress in the morning, choose clothing with fabric that thrills you. I love a good silk, but you might prefer something different. The only thing that matters is that the sensation on your skin is one that pleases you. While you eat breakfast, enjoy the warm mug of coffee or tea in your hand. Pet your cat or dog and delight in the feel of their fur. When you tuck your child in to sleep, run your hand down his arm and back and feel the softness of his skin. As you prepare for bed, rub your body lotion in slowly and enjoy the way it quenches your skin's thirst. By consciously enjoying touch today, you are recognizing that satisfaction comes from more than just the visual.

—→ 165 ←—

Concentrate on Taste

Today ⸺→ Concentrate on taste. Notice the zing of your toothpaste as you brush your teeth, the strength of your coffee as you sip, the flavor of your breakfast as you swallow, the sweetness of the fruit you bite into, the tanginess of the salad dressing at lunch, the sharpness of a hunk of cheese, the woodiness of your wine. Note all the flavors that come your way today. Being present as you eat or drink, savoring each taste, leads to even greater satisfaction.

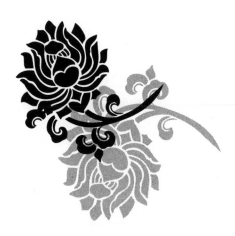

— 166 —

Concentrate on Sound

Today ⎯⎯ Concentrate on sound. In the morning, listen to the symphony of the birds as they awaken and call to each other. Notice the sound of the wind between trees, the hum of traffic in the middle distance, the drip of percolating coffee, the chatter of your children's voices, the noises you make while preparing breakfast, the click of your key in your car's ignition, the sound of your air conditioning or heater whirling to life, the cacophony of sounds in your office, the tap of your fingers on a keyboard, the din of activity at the gym, the ruckus of insects at nightfall. The sounds of the world can both calm and energize.

— 167 —

Concentrate on Smell

Today — Concentrate on smell. All day long, notice the scent of your soap, lotion, and perfume; your clothing, your breakfast, the front yard, traffic, your office space or school, your lunch, your dinner. Stop and smell the flowers on the side of the road, in your garden, or in the grocery store's flower buckets. Take a deep whiff of your child's scent or your partner's scent before going to bed. Savor the scents of your life.

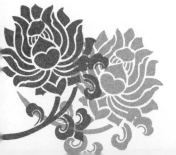

— 168 —

Concentrate on Sight

Today — Concentrate on sight. Take a long look out the window when you wake up. Choose an outfit that is visually interesting to you. Accessorize it in a way that pleases you visually. While traveling to work or school, turn off your iPod, cell phone, or radio, and take in the scenery around you. Make it a point to really look at the people you interact with today. Can you remember anything about what they are wearing or the expression on their face as they were talking to you? Relish the things you notice when you pay attention.

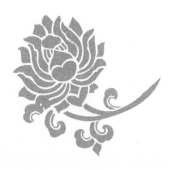

Put a Girl in Motion

I often lament what can only be described as my adult-onset athleticism. I didn't grow up an athlete. As much as I love sports, the powerful impact of Title IX didn't trickle down to me. But in my adulthood, I realized that my opportunities for athleticism were no longer determined by what sports my parents could afford to have me try or by what my school offered. My athleticism was in my own hands. I began lifting weights, running, rock climbing, cycling. I tried yoga, Pilates, surfing, and swimming. I became an athlete to the greatest extent that I was capable. My workouts have never been linked to my appearance; my body is my body, and it has no intentions of dramatically changing itself just because I run, bike, crunch, or lift. But the movement itself is therapeutic for me. Exercise provides sustenance for my body and mind that I can't get in any other form. Being physical is a gift that I believe women should be deliberate about embracing, and it's a gift that we should teach the girls in our lives to give themselves.

I was reminded of the joy and importance of empowering girls with the strength of their own bodies when board members from Circle de Luz, the nonprofit that was inspired by *Hijas Americanas,* took our Class of 2014 girls on a hike. We trekked through the state park for hours, the girls propelling themselves forward although none of them had ever been on a hike. Even when they realized the trail was longer then they had anticipated, they barreled ahead, motivated to finish. At our picnic lunch afterward, we told the girls that they had just completed five miles.

"If we had told you that we were going to hike five miles today, would you have thought you could do it?" I asked.

"No way" was the unanimous answer.

And yet, they did it. Over five miles of foot falls, they began to realize their power.

Today ——◦ Put a girl in motion. Have her join you for a hike, a long walk, a bike ride, a run, or a swim. Take her to your favorite yoga, Pilates, Zumba, or lifting class. Show her the strength of her body and the power of her mind. The more active our girls are, the more they realize the power they have, and the greater their confidence will be. Don't have a girl in your life? Check out the Women's Sports Foundation website (www.womenssports-foundation.org) to see if their GoGirlGo! program is being offered in a community near you.

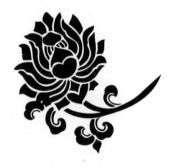

— 170 —

Listen to Your Intuition

How often have you said "I knew better than that!" after making a choice that had negative consequences? We are so much wiser than we are willing to believe, and that becomes especially true if our sense of self has been suffering. We need to build trust in ourselves.

Today —— Pay extra attention to your intuition. It knows what choice you should make. Whether that choice is about a relationship or some other big decision (to take the job or not, to move or to stay put), your intuition can probably tell you what's right. That said, we try to talk ourselves into things all the time, undermining our intuition. Call yourself on it when you find you are doing just that. Pay attention. Life keeps handing you the lesson you need to learn until you learn it.

— 171 —

Step Away from the Electronic Device

When I was teaching high school in the late nineties, my leadership students would always tell me, "You need to get a beeper or cell phone so we can get a hold of you when we need you." My answer to them was always really clear. *No.* "If you need me that much on a Wednesday night or a Saturday afternoon, then I have failed to do my job, which is to make you confident, independent, empowered thinkers."

Fast forward ten years and I have a PDA just like everyone else. I justify it because the sight of a full email inbox gives me anxiety. If I can just manage some of the mail as it comes in, then my life will ultimately be easier. Except there is an image that sticks in my mind from when I was still anti-cell phone; it moderates my Blackberry behavior and keeps the device from having a crack-like pull for me. I was walking to work on a beautiful spring day and a father and his young daughter were ahead of me on the sidewalk. He must have been walking her to preschool. He barked away on his cell phone, hung up, and then dropped her hand to type away on his PDA. Back on the cell phone, he barked some more. Off it again, he typed away. She looked up at him that entire walk, and never did he glance her way. He was living an entirely different life while her life passed before him. It is that image, that vision of the disconnected father, that keeps me from becoming too technologically tapped in.

Today —— Step away from your cell phone or PDA. Use them as sparingly as possible, and instead engage in the life that is right in front of your eyes. If you have a thirty-minute commute in the car, fight the urge to spend all thirty minutes talking on the phone just because you can. Turn on public radio or a station with music you can't resist. Look out the windows at the greenery that you pass. Think through different ways to solve a problem. Do anything but consume technology ad nauseum. While we believe that constantly checking email and voice mail will reduce our stress, research shows that it actually boosts it. When we begin to believe that our worth is determined by how quickly we respond to someone, by how fast we process technology, we lose the true sense of our worth—which isn't in processing but in being. Each time we allow someone else to suggest that we should be working when we are technically supposed to be off of work, we give away the power we have over our own lives. So go on a no-PDA, no-cell-phone fast for today and then put yourself on a diet (this time a diet is okay!) for the days to come. Designate a few times during the day to read and respond to messages and enjoy the control you regain over your own life.

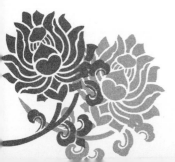

— 172 —

Assert Yourself

A re you the person who gives in or never says a word in one (or all) of your relationships? Standing up for yourself in a way that is appropriate for the situation allows you to express your needs without being disrespectful or making demands. While being assertive shouldn't devalue the other person involved in the conversation, it should give value to you and what you are thinking, feeling, and experiencing. By making your own viewpoints known, you are placing value on your perspective.

Today —— Be assertive when the situation calls for it. Maybe someone kept you waiting for a meeting or let you down in another way. Use the facts and avoid blame ("I scheduled our meeting from 1:00 PM until 2:00 PM, and there are other things I have to attend to right at two, so I just wanted to let you know that we only have twenty-five minutes to discuss our strategy on this issue") to make your case. The goal is not to have everything change immediately, but for you to give voice to your experience, thus valuing your perspective.

Go to a Museum

I first visited a museum on a school field trip. I remember walking through the Columbia Museum of Art (where I would have my wedding reception so many years later), mesmerized by the paintings that showed beauty in so many different manifestations. Museums show the range of what should imprint in our mind's eye, and they show us possibility.

Today —— Visit an art museum. As you take in the exhibits, look at the various images that depict women throughout history—real and imagined—and notice how there isn't just one standard of beauty in the world of art. Since art, indeed, imitates life, walk away feeling the impact of that vast display of beauty.

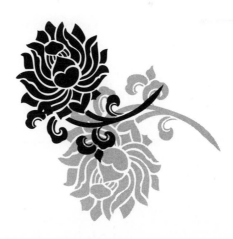

Develop an "I Have Decided" Approach

Three words can be so very effective: *I have decided*. I have decided... that I am going to be a published writer one day. I have decided... that I will be healthy. I have decided... that I will be an artist. I have decided... that I will not fear x or y or z. "I have decided" acknowledges the journey and process that we all must undertake to get the things (experiences, joys, etc.) we most want, while also acknowledging the power we have to make it happen.

Today —— Write an "I have decided" statement in your *Beautiful You* journal. Why did you make this decision and how will you accomplish it? Consider writing an "I have decided" statement in your *Beautiful You* journal every day as you develop your personal vision and sense of self. Perhaps the statement will be the same some days and totally different on others, but it should always be about owning your own power.

— 175 —

Go Dry

Sometimes we self-medicate with food. Sometimes we self-medicate with alcohol. Over the years, I've had several friends go dry, sometimes of their own volition and sometimes because others have suggested it. What they learned about themselves in the process was that drinking kept them from feeling what they needed to feel, addressing what they needed to address, and growing in the ways they needed to grow.

That's not necessarily true for every person who enjoys a great stout or fine wine, but it is true that some people use alcohol in order to keep from feeling things. If alcohol is getting in the way of your being able to celebrate your brilliance, the only way through is to learn to stop using alcohol as a crutch.

Today —— Whether or not you suspect you use alcohol as a crutch, take a break from it today. Just see how not having it makes you feel, and what thinking about "going dry" unveils for you.

DAY

— 176 —

Break Your Addictions

Maybe one of your dependencies is alcohol, maybe it's something else—a different substance, the need to always be connected to others, some other particular behavior. Addictions are a hazard to living full, happily realized lives because they keep us disconnected from what we really think and feel. They can paralyze us and prevent us from taking action. The first step in breaking an addiction is examining whether or not we have a dependency, something that slows us down or dulls us from being who we are meant to be.

Today ⟶ In your *Beautiful You* journal, consider whether or not you have any dependencies that get in the way of fully becoming your best self. Is there a crutch you use to manage experiences you aren't fully prepared to manage on your own? When and why did this dependency begin? What has it done for you? How has it limited you? What would you do without it? What would be a good first step in your efforts to decrease the presence of this dependency in your life?

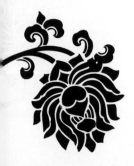

— 177 —

Choose Rejuvenation

There is nothing more life affirming than choosing to do something—even something small—that provides your soul with a sense of rejuvenation. For some women that might be a manicure. For others, it's a massage. For still others, it might be a run through the park or an afternoon reading in the sunshine. Whatever it is, if it adds to your sense of well-being—if it makes your soul happy—it is worthwhile.

Today —— Do something that helps you feel rejuvenated. You can't do everything you want to do every single day, but just for today you can do one small thing that will boost your sense of well-being by addressing your own needs.

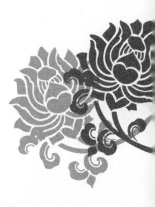

— 178 —

Make a Greatest Hits List

We sometimes lose focus of how far we've come and how much we've accomplished. Being reminded of our successes and victories grounds us in our competence and abilities.

Today ——— Take out your *Beautiful You* journal and make a list of the successes you have enjoyed throughout your life. At what moments have you felt especially proud of yourself? Capture as many of them as you can in your journal so you can see the magnitude of your successes and revisit this list when you want to check your progress. Later, as you remember other successes or do more things, add to the list.

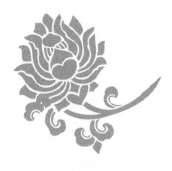

— 179 —

Tell Your Secret

We so often bury things, thinking that our secrets are so shameful that giving them voice would only give them power. In fact, the opposite is true. Telling a secret lessens its power; shame dies with the secret's liberation. Most experiences seem more manageable once they have been shared with a trusted friend, a family member, or a therapist who is likely to offer you much-needed support. When you share a secret, you announce that it no longer has power over you. Inevitably, you also find out that many other people share your "secret" experiences, and they often have insights or possible solutions that you can try. The power truly becomes yours.

Today —— Tell one of your secrets rather than continuing to suffer in silence. Being heard and using your voice are wonderful catalysts to confidence.

— 180 —

Contribute

One of my greatest joys is contributing my resources—both financial and practical—to causes I believe in. When I know that something I do benefits others, I feel especially empowered and inspired. This isn't just true for me. Being generous boosts everyone's happiness and sense of well-being because it reminds us that the world is not just ours—it's not only about us. It also reminds us that contributing leads to positive outcomes for everyone involved.

Today ⟞ Choose an amount that feels generous to you (but doesn't break your bank) and donate to a local cause that has meaning for you. Even if you send this group an annual donation, open up your checkbook today and send something their way. Don't know where to donate? Visit the web site of your local United Way to learn about nonprofits in your area that might be doing work that really speaks to you. Go to www.liveunited.org to get started.

— 181 —

Think About What You Don't Think About

I read Naomi Wolff's *The Beauty Myth* years ago. And all these years later I use a few chapters of it in the body image class I teach. What I like my students to consider is Wolff's theory is that by culturally fixating on thinness and beauty in women, we keep our women bound, unable to reach their full prominence. The "beauty myth," if you will, is more about keeping women obedient than beautiful.

But why would men—or the establishment—want to keep women obedient? a student will often ask. Why does it matter? It matters, I tell them, because power and possibility would profoundly change if women weren't bound—even in theory—in some way.

Today —— In your *Beautiful You* journal, consider what your biggest concern would be if it weren't your body or some other part of yourself. Where would you devote your energy? What would you be hell-bent on changing? Now that you know what you would be thinking about if you weren't thinking about beauty standards and body ideals, what will you do with that knowledge?

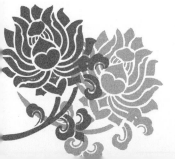

— 182 —

Create a Budget

lright, I know what some of you are thinking. What does money have to do with self-confidence and a positive sense of self? As it turns out, a lot. When we spend wildly and let our expenses get out of control, we're indicating a need to self-medicate through consuming. Moreover, we are revealing that we aren't really taking charge of ourselves—we're operating from an impulsive, insecure place that only fosters more impulsiveness and insecurity. By creating a budget, we signal to our inner self that we are in control, that we have a plan for today and the future, and that we understand the difference between wants and needs and have given each their proper due by creating a system that allows us to act deliberately when it comes to money.

Today — Create a budget that reflects your fixed expenses and your living expenses that might be variable, like groceries and savings. Have you tried budgeting in the past only to not have it work? Consider hiring a financial advisor or asking a friend or sibling who has those skills to share her insights with you. By taking control of your money, you are exercising confidence in being in charge of yourself.

— 183 —

Change Your Language

At the end of each semester, I ask students in my body image seminar to write a process paper, a final paper that details their processing of the semester's classroom experience. The papers are always fascinating, and they often give me new insights.

A recent process paper started with the following passage:

"I have dealt with an eating disorder for eight years now. I am careful to say "I have dealt with" and not "I have" an eating disorder because I'd like to think it's an obstacle, not a commitment. Saying I have an eating disorder suggests that it is something that I own and is a part of me. But it's not. . . . I don't own it. I deal with it. I refuse to let it define me."

What I loved about that passage was its thoughtfulness. Language is so important. What we own, what we have, what we face, those can all be such different things, have such different connotations. Owning our language and, thus, the implications of that language, can be so empowering. It can show that we define ourselves rather than allow ourselves to be defined. And changing our language can often be the very first step in changing our minds.

Today —— In your *Beautiful You* journal, consider the language that you use and how it limits your self-definition. What are things you say that limit your possibilities? How can you change your language to change your mind?

Shop at a Farmers Market

Shopping at the local farmers market brings me so much joy. I visit with neighbors while relishing the beautiful produce and joyful entertainment that are always in abundance at my local market. I am exposed to new fruits and vegetables that I take home to try; just this past year, I learned how to prepare edamame and kale. I enjoy the taste of just-off-the-farm produce so much that I am encouraged to eat a more healthy diet. I cherish the fact that I am doing something that is both good for my soul (all that friendly, warm human contact), my body (all those lovely, healthy, mostly organic fruits and veggies), and my community (buying local and supporting the small-town farmer).

Today —— Shop at a local farmers market. Buy a fruit or vegetable you have never tried and ask the farmer for suggestions on how to prepare it. When it's time to eat, savor the taste and your success!

Realize That Before the Media Can Fully Change, We Need to Change

I used to think all that needed to happen to improve our collective body image and self-esteem was for the media to change. What I have realized, though, is that we need to change first. The media gives us what we ask for, what we respond to, and what we keep revisiting. Media companies have profits to make, so giving us what we want is a very wise strategy. But we need to tell the media we want something different. Our tastes and tolerances have to change in order for the messages we receive to change.

Today —— In your *Beautiful You* journal, consider how your media tastes perpetuate standards that make you uncomfortable. Do you buy countless celebrity magazines, sending the message that celebrities' lives and bodies—and not just their work—should be up for grabs? Do you watch programs that exploit, debase, demean, or send negative messages? How can you change so that our media changes?

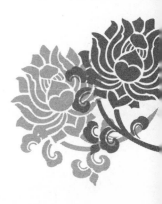

— 186 —

Take a Bath

Watching my baby boy splash through bath time reminds me of the joy of doing even the most mundane of tasks—like getting our bodies clean—at a leisurely pace.

Today ——— Treat your mind and body to at least a twenty-minute bath. Feel free to just shut your eyes for a little meditation, to read, or to sip a cup of tea. Maybe you'll use some fancy soaps that you were given months (years!) ago.

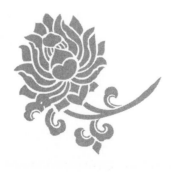

— 187 —

Ask Someone

ave you ever noticed how one slight change in our appearance—a zit here, a gray hair there, a tiny expression line—becomes monumental in our own eyes? We talk to someone after we notice the offense, and all we can think is, *She's staring at that zit on my nose.* Meanwhile, the truth is that the person you're talking to has not even noticed your zit. Really, we are a lot less critical of others than we are of ourselves.

Today —— Get some perspective. Ask someone you speak to on a regular basis if she notices anything different about you and then consider her answer. No one else fixates on our perceived flaws the way we do.

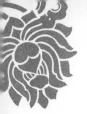

— 188 —

Change Your Wish

Maybe you have spent years wishing for something: good hair, clear skin, a thin frame, silky locks, whiter teeth, whatever. But is that really what you want?

A woman I know said recently, "I used to say I wish I had good skin, but in reality, the only thing I wish for is to be accepted by society as another form of beautiful."

When we wish for happiness to be accessible to us only after we have changed ourselves—sometimes in ways that aren't even possible—the possibility for happiness isn't just fleeting, it's a torturing tease.

Today —— Change your wish. What if what you wished for was to be considered enough—in all ways—just as you are? Treat yourself with compassion.

— 189 —

Take No Hostages

I have watched episodes from the various seasons of *The Biggest Loser* over the years, and I am always struck by how the participants talk about "getting their lives back" when they describe the effects of their weight loss. Yet I don't think that change comes only because they shed pounds.

The reality is that when we are consumed with thinking about our bodies—with being embarrassed of our bodies, no matter our size—we are being held hostage. And when we are held hostage, our soul suffers. We get softer, less dynamic, more frail. We lose our way. We quit living life to its fullest. Sometimes we barely live it at all.

Today —— Realize that when your body holds you hostage, it dampens your spirit and tampers with your soul. Today, give yourself room to grow and blossom.

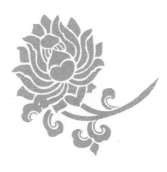

— 190 —

Talk to Your Partner about Your Anxieties

In my body image seminar, I ask students to conduct body image interviews. They interview two different people in their lives about their experiences with self-esteem and body image. Their final product is a paper that examines what the students learned about the people they interviewed, what they think shaped those people's views, and how the things they learned in the interviews has affected their own ideas about self-image and body issues.

Sometimes students interview their boyfriends or girlfriends. And these students often say that the interviews, motivated by a school assignment, resulted in some of the most honest conversations about insecurities and confidence they've ever had with their partners. They realize how much they've avoided discussing these things in their relationships, and how avoidance actually built up their insecurities and decreased the pleasure they could be finding in their partnerships. Many of the students concluded that they could tackle their own insecurities and anxieties by unveiling them, and they resolved to move forward differently in their relationships.

Today —— Talk to your partner about an anxiety you have so you can move past insecurity and toward self-acceptance and self-assurance. Don't have a partner? Call the friend that you have identified as your go-to girl and share your thoughts with her.

— 191 —

Let Shame or Guilt Go

Maybe someone has gone beyond silent criticism. Maybe someone has made his or her thoughts known. Today is the day to let go of the feelings those negative opinions elicited.

Today —— Jot down things you've been told about how your body should look or be in this world. Write each statement on a separate piece of paper. Now light a candle and burn each statement. Next, affirm yourself by asserting that no one has the right to tell you what you should look like or how you should be in this world. All that matters is that you are empowered to make those choices for yourself.

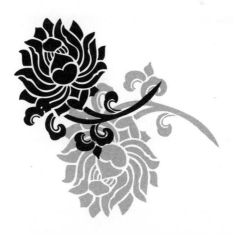

— 192 —

Lift Weights

For four months before we brought our baby boy home, I lifted weights four times a week for forty-five minutes each time. I wasn't concerned with how my biceps looked, but I was concerned with how they functioned. I knew that on the day I met my baby boy, I would instantly need to be able to carry at least fifteen extra pounds, and that I'd be carrying that weight around almost all of the time. The best way for me to prepare for that new physical challenge was by practicing for it almost every day.

Becoming stronger also boosted my self-confidence. I could carry my suitcases filled with books for signings without a problem, lift them into an overhead compartment on an airplane without hesitation, and then help someone else with his or her bag without worrying about losing control and knocking someone in the head. Knowing that I have the strength required to meet my own needs is incredibly empowering.

Today —— Consult with a fitness trainer about a weight-training plan that will work for you, take a strength-training class at your gym, or check out a fitness DVD at your local library. Not comfortable going it alone? Ask an experienced friend to show you a thing or two about lifting weights.

— 193 —

Shine a Light

A few years ago, I came across an incredible-smelling candle. Until that day, I could take or leave candles. I thought of them as an extravagant way to spend some dollars (and I still think they can be). But then someone gave me a passion fruit–scented candle as a hostess gift. When I lit it, it filled the room and my heart with the scent of pleasure and happiness. Now I savor those passion fruit candles. While I tend to light them only on rainy or gray days, my mood lifts as soon as I catch a whiff of that scent. Sometimes, all we need is a little sensory stimulation to lighten or brighten our mood.

Today —— Find a candle that smells fabulous and light it as a treat for yourself.

— 194 —

Focus on Listening

Sometimes we get so self-conscious about what we have to offer that we don't even offer people what they most need: a good listener.

I was in the car today, talking to my best friend from childhood, and she told me that her Grandma died.

"Jenny, I am so sorry," I told her, and she began to tell me about the last few days, their sad moments and sweet ones too.

We started talking about crying, and she shared such a valuable insight about it. When you give someone a Kleenex, she said, it's like telling them that they have grieved enough and that they should clean themselves up and move on. It's better, she shared, to let them ask for it, so they don't feel like they are being given a subtle or not so subtle message.

"Sometimes," my sweet, wise friend said, "it is okay to just sit and listen. You don't have to know just what to say."

Today —— Concentrate on being a better listener. Watch every single conversation today and hold yourself back from cutting anyone off. Quit worrying about your point and all the parts of it while the other person is talking. Just listen. Maintain eye contact with the person rather than allowing yourself to be distracted. Nod, smile, show visual interest, touch a hand, and give soft verbal cues that you understand. All of these techniques will really help you hear what is being said. Being a better listener allows you to be a better friend, coworker, parent, or partner, and being any of these things to the best of your ability boosts your sense of well-being.

— 195 —

Reflect on Your Strength

Sometimes we lose touch with our story. In August 2008, my husband and I thought we would adopt a baby sometime in 2010. And then, one Friday afternoon that same month, we learned of a baby boy whose mother could not care for him, and we knew he was our son. The decision was made in an instant. The feeling that he was our son was so clear.

But just two days later, I awoke with a palpable discomfort. I went out on our front porch, sat on a swing that a friend had carefully built for us as a wedding present, and I wept. At first, I wept for this baby boy and his mother. At the imbalance of wealth in this world and how reconciling it seems enormous and daunting. I wept at this mama's love for her child, at her bravery and her vision for him, and her unselfishness. I wept at the enormous responsibility we had to her if we were to become his parents. I wept about whether or not we could be the stewards she and her boy deserved. Then I wept because I wondered if it was terribly selfish to bring an African child to the United States, where he might encounter racial bias in a way that does not even have words in his native country. I wept because I wondered if we were naive to think that love and effort and care were enough to give an African child the life he deserves here. I wept because I knew what it was like to be judged for being "other," what it was like to be denied for being other, what it was like to be spit at for being other. I worried that we might be complicit in subjecting a child to a life that would not be impoverished in the traditional sense but would be impoverished in another sense, one that was just as crucial to his development. Finally, I called one of my dearest friends and told her about this anxiety of mine. How I did not want to do more harm than good. How I did not want to be naive. And her words to me were like a salve.

"What if your whole life—everything you have experienced up to this point, your own personal experiences of being the other, your bicultural background, your major in African American studies, your work with African American boys, your teaching so many young people of various backgrounds, your work capturing the stories of Latinas so that they could have a voice and a vehicle for expression in the mainstream—what if all of that was simply your dress rehearsal for this, for being this boy's mom?"

My friend helped remind me of who I was and what I had gone through. She helped me see that the the challenges I'd weathered had given me character that would now serve as a compass for how we parented our baby boy. I had lost touch with my story for a moment, but she brought me back to it and helped me understand that the strength I had in me was enough.

Today —— In your *Beautiful You* journal, write about the times in your life where you took a situation that was difficult and navigated it in a way that was successful. Yes, getting back on the bike after wiping out in front of everyone in the neighborhood when you were six counts. Reflecting on your brave and powerful moments will give you perspective, self-assurance, and confidence.

— 196 —

Go Without Makeup

I like putting on makeup as much as the next girl. My can't-do-without product? Blush. It seems the name Rosie has inspired my desire to always sport a flush. But we can become too dependent on our "made-up" looks which, if we aren't careful, can make us feel dissatisfied with our real skin.

Today —— Give your skin—and yourself—a breather. Go without makeup. Realize that your identity is rooted in your soul, not your rouged cheeks or mascara-enhanced lashes.

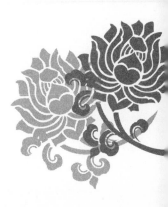

— 197 —

Don't Lose Sleep Over Finding Mr. or Ms. Right

Too often, we place the possibility of our own happiness in someone else's hands. We think, *If he loves me, then I will be happy*, or *If she notices me, then I will be fulfilled*. That is way too much personal power to be giving away to someone else. We need to take back the power we give away so easily and understand that the way to our own happiness is through self-love.

Today —— Mentally say goodbye forever to the "one who got away" and drop the search for "the one." Instead, spend time with the one who is always there–you. Far too many women have lost themselves on the journey to coupledom. Lose yourself, instead, in the journey to yourself.

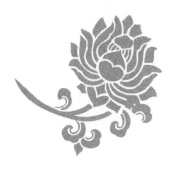

— 198 —

Write Yourself a Letter

My Masters in Fine Arts program was a low-residency model. We would start each semester on campus in Vermont, where for just under two weeks we'd attend lectures, workshops, and readings in an intensive 9:00 AM to 9:00 PM format. When the residency ended, we would gather for a closing ceremony before we returned to our respective homes for fifteen weeks of work done on our own, sent in to our advisors on regular three-week intervals. At the closing ceremony, back in Vermont, one of the final exercises was letter writing. Pens, paper, and envelopes made their way around our circle, and we were instructed to write letters to a few people in the program and—did I hear that right?—a letter to ourselves that would be mailed out to us later by on-campus staff members.

Write a letter to myself? Not so much. So I addressed letters to my roommates and other friends in the program, and for the first semester or two, that was it. Finally, I softened a bit and wrote a letter to myself, then promptly forgot about it. What a surprise it was months later to check the mailbox and see my own handwriting.

"What's this?" I thought. It wasn't until I had unfolded the paper that I realized this was the letter I had written to myself, a letter designed to cheer on my efforts at writing my final manuscript while working full-time. It gave me a much-needed boost by reminding me of my determination.

Today —— Write yourself a letter that celebrates who you are and where you are going. Then put it in an envelope, address it, and give it to someone you trust to mail it to you when she thinks it is time.

— 199 —

Use a Salt Scrub

A person can get so good at ignoring her body that she ignores its needs and denies it any sensual pleasure. Yet caring for your body is a wonderful way to express gratitude for it, while also meeting some of its needs.

Today ⸺ Revitalize your skin by using a commercial salt scrub, or mix your own scrub by combining sea salt and an essential oil in equal parts. Apply the scrub to your body; rub it over each area, using gentle, circular motions, until the skin flushes. After you are done, soak in a warm tub before rinsing off the remainder of the solution.

— 200 —

Realize That You Should Be Cared For By You

I became incredibly ill during my third year of teaching. Determined to keep my illness from interfering with my life or the lives of my students, I ignored the symptoms for as long as I possibly could before finally seeing a doctor. The diagnosis of hypoglycemia took months. Once we realized that my blood sugar was strikingly low, I was only willing to correct my food behaviors. Although stress was an aggravating factor in my illness, I could not stop working hard because, in my mind, if I stopped giving as much as I was giving, one of my kids would suffer. And I could not have that.

That spring, I found myself at the doctor's office during my planning period, trying to quickly get a prescription to temper the illness that plagued me. "You have bronchitis," my doctor told me, "and an ear infection and tonsillitis." He scribbled a prescription out for an antibiotic, and I raced to the local pharmacy, counting the minutes until I needed to be back at school for my next class. At the pharmacy, I approached the counter, with cash and my prescription stuffed into the pockets of my khakis. I left my purse, which contained my driver's license, in the car. As I moved toward that counter, I felt the world spin and then the lights went out.

I awoke to see a brigade of firemen, the first responders to the 911 call made by the pharmacists, above me.

"We need an ambulance for Jane Doe," one of them said into a radio. I checked out again for a moment and then came back.

"I know my name," I offered, and so they tagged my information into the system and then loaded me into the arriving ambulance.

At the hospital, a young doctor oversaw my care. How did I get so sick, he wondered. I offered what I knew.

"You work too much," he said. "You have to change that."

I didn't. A week later, I was back in the emergency room, this time coughing up blood, and the same doctor was there.

"I am willing to keep seeing you here," he said, "if you are willing to keep landing yourself here. But I want to believe that you are smarter than that, and that you will do what you need to do to stay out of here."

I decided to listen that time.

Today —— Begin to develop the radical conviction that you should be cared for by you.

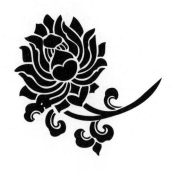

Identify Your Excuses

here are likely things you wanted to accomplish in the past that you didn't. There will always be barriers to our progress, but knowing what the barriers are helps us better understand which ones we really have no control over—and which ones we are allowing to control us.

Today ⟶ In your *Beautiful You* journal, answer these questions. What goals have you wanted to accomplish that have yet to be accomplished? What is holding you back? Do you have more control than you realized in the past?

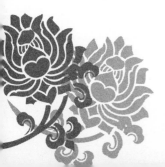

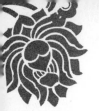

— 202 —

Create a Daily Skincare Regimen

One of the most decadent parts of my day comes at the very end, when I walk into my bathroom, wash my face, and rub moisturizing cream all over my skin. It feels indulgent and my skin swallows the moisture in gulps, gratefully. That little bit of self-care allows me to take a moment for myself while enjoying a simple pleasure. It also makes me understand that my body's happiness is quite literally in my hands.

Today —— Create a simple daily skincare regimen that caters to your skincare and personal needs. Bask in those simple moments of self-care.

⊶ 203 ⊷

Just Be with Someone

Too often when we are with people we care about, we aren't fully present. We are distracted by the television, the cell phone, the computer, the PDA, the newspaper. When we bypass the chance to fully engage with someone, we bypass the sense of well-being and meaning that interpersonal connection could have provided us. And when we rob our experiences of meaning, we lose our capacity to root and ground ourselves.

Today ⟶ Be with someone for thirty minutes without doing anything else (eating a meal together is okay, but no other multitasking efforts allowed). Enjoy the company, camaraderie, and perspective you gain by just being with someone else.

— 204 —

Revel In What Is Important

I read an interview with the actor Michael J. Fox, who has Parkinson's disease. In it, he revealed that one of the changes in his approach to life post-diagnosis is that when his kids say, "Dad, come look at this," or "do this," etc., he drops what he is doing and responds, rather than saying, "Just a second." What is most important to him right now is his family—enjoying his family members and allowing them to enjoy him. By getting up and going to them when he is called, he is reveling in what's most important to him.

Today —— Consider this. Life is so much more fleeting than we realize. Days can seem long when we are in the midst of them, but when we look back at them, it's as if they passed in a flash. Open up your *Beautiful You* journal and answer this question: What is really, really important to you? Now consider how you can live in a way that honors the importance that has in your life.

— 205 —

Write a Letter

I t had been a hell of a day. I walked up the stairs to my apartment slowly, painfully, wanting nothing more than to erase the amount of trouble that two kids from my first period class had gotten into. I felt guilty because they only knew each other thanks to my seating chart. Separate, they were two bright kids on their way to success. Together, they were two kids latched so hard to each other they were drowning. Inside the apartment, I kicked back on the couch and started sorting the mail: bills, catalogs; nothing of consequence, it seemed, until I came upon a cream-colored, hand-addressed envelope. There was no return address. I ripped it open and found a touching, anonymous note inside. The writer told me that he or she was thinking of me, remembering things I had done to inspire him or her, celebrating who I was, and wishing me well. The note ended without a signature. I had no idea who sent it, but on a day where I felt like I was anything but inspirational, a mysterious someone had unknowingly refilled my well.

Today —— Write a letter to someone who has touched your life. Talk about the difference this person has made to you and what you most appreciate about him or her. Then drop that gift of love in the mail. In just a few days, you'll buoy that person's self-esteem. But the positive effect of celebrating someone else should instantly buoy your own.

— 206 —

Designate a Happiness Spot

As soon as I was done reading that sweet note from the anonymous sender, I knew exactly what I would do with it. The year before, I had purchased a beautiful wooden writing box that came with a stand and occupied a corner of my bedroom. Inside, a tray held stamps and note cards. Below it, the open box was the perfect storage site for letters and cards that really spoke to me and that I couldn't bear to throw out. The box also offered the perfect remedy to a bad day. Whenever I felt blue or questioned my worth, I would sit down beside it, pop open the top, and reach blindly inside. Whatever I pulled out—a birthday card from five years ago or a recent note from a student—always reminded me of who I was at my core and how fortunate I was.

Today —⁓ Designate a happiness box, drawer, or envelope. Go through the sentimental items you have collected over time and put the things that most lift your spirit in your new happiness spot. When you need a boost of inspiration, return to your happiness spot to bask in your brilliance.

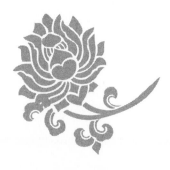

— 207 —

Create a Happiness Spot in Your Inbox

Years after I ended my teaching career, a familiar name popped up in my email inbox. A former student had written me a lovely note, thanking me for what I had taught her and for making her feel like she was seen. I realized this email was like the anonymous handwritten letter I had received back when I was teaching. Wanting to hold onto it, I quickly created an email inbox folder labeled PERSONAL, where I could save this email and others like it.

Today ——— Create an inbox folder for emails that celebrate you. Name it BEAUTIFUL ME, CELEBRATIONS, BRILLIANCE, or even PERSONAL. Now begin using it to store electronic celebrations of yourself. Whenever you need a boost while you are working at the computer, open up your file and read away.

— 208 —

Realize That You Are Created for a Unique Purpose

The wonder of humanity is that we are each unique, and it is our uniqueness that makes us beautiful and valuable. You are here for a unique purpose, a purpose only you can fulfill. There is no one else who shares your particular combination of DNA and unique experiences, no one else who has the same talents you do.

Today — Focus on what makes you unique and on what purpose you have in this world. Concentrate on what you have to give as the person you are today.

— 209 —

Consider What You Find Beautiful

I f we have lived for too long with a critical eye toward beauty, especially our own beauty, we can lose our ability to even notice it. Taking delight in the beauty that is inside you, and the beauty that surrounds you every day, is an essential step in celebrating your brilliance.

Today ⟶ Answer this question in your *Beautiful You* journal. What did you find beautiful today?

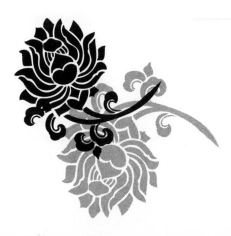

⫸ 210 ⫷

Watch a Foreign Film

One of the things I am struck by every time I watch a foreign film is the great variety of styles and looks represented by women around the world. It is a refreshing reminder that beauty is vast and varied, despite the fact that we are fed a very narrow standard of beauty by the American media.

Today ⫸ Watch a foreign film that features women prominently so you can shake up your own visual routine. Some options include *Run Lola Run, Whale Rider, Once, Ma Vie En Rose, Slumdog Millionaire, Y Tu Mamá También,* and *Crouching Tiger, Hidden Dragon.*

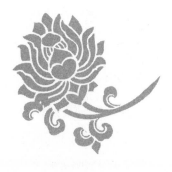

—— 211 ——

Realize Your Good Fortune

My family settled in the United States when I was two years old, when my dad received his final posting in the U.S. Army. We moved to Columbia, South Carolina (don't crinkle your nose—it's a great small city!), where we lived on Fort Jackson before moving off the military base when I was in first grade. The next year, my dad retired from the Army. Not long after, while I was still working my way through elementary school, my brother and sister graduated from high school. With my brother and sister done with their secondary educations, my parents toyed with the idea of moving back to Puerto Rico with me. I toyed with ideas of how to keep the suitcases from coming off the shelves and the FOR SALE signs out of the yard. Ultimately, they decided to stay in the United States; largely, I think, because they knew I would be afforded a better education and opportunity here.

That decision had a greater impact on me than my parents could have ever imagined. It was the sacrifice of their lives, really, to choose my education over being with their families. My decisions as a young adult often came from knowing deep inside what they had done for me. I wasn't the kid who pushed the envelope with her parents. I didn't talk back. I recognized that if something about living here was hard for them—finding work, finding respect, finding a fair wage for their skills—they were dealing with that difficulty because they chose to stay here for me. I gave them grace because they gave me opportunity. I developed an incredible sense of responsibility when some teenagers were nursing an incredible self-consciousness. The extent of my good fortune has continued to be never far from my mind.

Today —— Consider your life. In your *Beautiful You* journal, reflect on what have been your moments of good fortune. What have those moments offered you?

Create a Memory Board

Memories of joyful moments can lift our spirits and put us back in touch with our centers.

Today ⟶ Create a memory board to display in your home or office, complete with photos, ticket stubs, cards, or other mementos that help you get back in touch with your most genuine self. Want to do something a little different? One of my friends has a wire garland with stars hung in her office. She uses novelty clothesline clips to hang her mementos on the garland and turns to it every time she needs a smile or some centering.

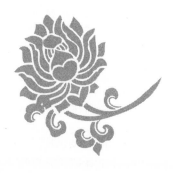

— 213 —

Pass Something On

In the summer of 2008, one of my dearest friends lost her father. He was a man who was adored—by her, by me, by many. He had been battling cancer, and my friend, her brother, and their families were able to spend the last two months of his life with him, honoring his life while it was still being lived. When I heard the news, I booked my ticket to be with her, my heart broken open in sympathy. My father had battled cancer just a few years earlier, and I remember how I felt as I drove the highway between my home and his chemotherapy treatment center every few weeks; how scared I was of living without my father. I didn't know if I could exist in a world without my dad. I didn't know who to be if I wasn't my father's daughter. Boarding the plane to be with my dear friend, I knew that she was facing what I most feared.

As I sat by her side on the evening after the funeral, she talked about her fears. Instinctively, my hands went to my neck and fingered the necklace I wore. I had purchased it a year before, a simple silver plate with the word fearlessness stamped across it. Without thinking, I took it off and put it on my friend. The necklace had served me well. It was time for her to have it.

A few weeks later, feeling naked without a reminder around my neck of who I was or wanted to be, I purchased another fearlessness necklace. A few months later, a young woman I knew came to me during an incredibly difficult time in her life. Instinctively, I thought of the necklace and turned it over to her.

"Are you sure?" she responded. "I can't take this from you."

"You need it right now," I told her. "And when you no longer need it, I want you to pass it on to a person in your life who does."

Today — Think about the people in your life and the things in your life. Is there something that you have right now that no longer serves you as powerfully as it once did but could be an important memento or reminder in the life of someone you love? If so, pass it on. You will be practicing letting go while meaningfully building a bond with someone else, taking an important step in your journey to find yourself.

— 214 —

Find Your Signature Piece

My interest in necklaces that make a statement or serve as a reminder started in my mid-twenties, when I began to travel. After a month in Brazil, where I worked with ten students and another leader to build a healthcare clinic and dig wells, our hosts gave us necklaces with red-eyed frog charms on them. Later, wearing that necklace reminded me of our time in Brazil and the woman I had grown into while I was there. Many times, lost in thought, I'd find myself fingering the frog around my neck. When I'd realize what I was doing, I'd remember the lessons I wanted to hold onto from my experience in Brazil.

Years later, my signature necklace became a brightly colored globe with the words "Brave Heart" on one side and "Happy Life" on the other. It reminded me to be both grateful and strong. My next signature piece was the fearlessness necklace. Made by Me&Ro, proceeds from the necklace benefit the Joyful Heart Foundation, a nonprofit organization dedicated to healing, educating, and empowering survivors of sexual assault, domestic violence, and child abuse. Today, my signature necklace is a silver globe with a six-point-star cutout designed by Mary Alice Mitchell, a silver artist in my community. Mary Alice contributed her skills to creating necklaces that benefit Circle de Luz, the nonprofit I was inspired to start after writing and promoting *Hijas Americanas: Beauty, Body Image, and Growing Up Latina*. What I love about having a signature piece is that it is centering, a visible reminder of who I am. When my fingers move to my neck in thought, when someone mentions the necklace in conversation, or when I look in the mirror while washing my hands, the reminder grounds me, which is helpful in a world that often throws me off balance.

Today —— Look through your jewelry to see if you already own your signature piece. Maybe it is a gift your parents gave you when you were twelve, or a piece your grandmother handed down to you. If you don't yet own a signature piece, look for that bracelet, ring, or necklace that gives you just the right message. Try www.etsy.com for a one-of-a-kind handmade piece or even something with a powerful message.

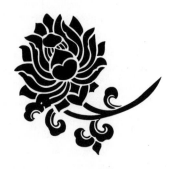

DAY

— 215 —

Consider Your Aspirations

How do you know when to keep going toward something, whether it will bring you the happiness and self-satisfaction that you have believed it might?

For years, Karen Williams practiced law as a profession and practiced yoga on the side. Over time, the satisfaction she received from yoga began to outpace that generated by her law career. The desire to create a wellness center, complete with yoga, meditation, and other wellness services, became a plan rather than a fantasy. But moving from corporate attorney to wellness center owner would prove to be a considerable journey—one that would require concluding a lucrative professional career, purchasing and transforming an existing business, finding and renovating an adequate business space, managing staff and student expectations, and developing an entirely new set of complex skills…from accounting and marketing to website design and more. It would take not weeks or months, but years to accomplish.

So, Williams began walking the arduous path of making her dream a reality. Periodically, doubt, exhaustion, or difficult practicalities would distract her from the tasks at hand. When they did, she asked herself a simple question: Is this a worthy aspiration? Because the answer was always a resounding "Yes!" She knew that things would fall into place, even on the very hardest days. That question continues to serve Williams, who is now the owner of Centered Wellness in Charlotte, North Carolina, for professional and personal matters alike. If the aspiration is a worthy one, there is freedom to run fast and fly high…without fear. If the aspiration is a worthy one, obstacles will be temporary and impermanent, and even the most tremendous of goals becomes attainable.

Today —— What possibilities—either personal or professional—have been weighing on your mind lately? Now ask yourself the question, "Are these worthy aspirations?" If the answer is a resounding yes, do exactly what Williams did. Go. Run. It is when we align ourselves with what we want most that our joy and beauty truly flourishes.

— 216 —

Focus Your Day

My best days come when I deliberately choose to focus. By purposefully thinking about what I want to accomplish and what I want to enjoy or gain from a day, I am both productive and treat myself well. Unfortunately, I have found that I don't treat myself well automatically. It takes planning and discipline to give myself the life I imagine every day. By focusing myself each day, I take greater pleasure in my life and feel a greater sense of well-being.

Today — Consider your long-term dreams. Then, in your *Beautiful You* journal, consider what will help you, today, achieve a sense of well-being and harmony with your dreams, and set that small goal. A series of these smaller steps allows you to see the effort you are making toward your greater well-being while giving you a sense of accomplishment and satisfaction today. By enjoying your journey, you are allowing every day to be a part of your accomplishment.

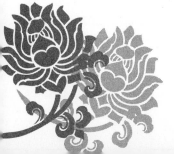

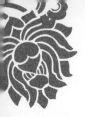

— 217 —

Don't Be Afraid To Reach Out to a Stranger

Sometimes our biggest dreams are exactly that: dreams. We don't know enough about the idea to take action, and yet it keeps holding our interest. When that happens, I find it helps to reach out to someone who can teach you something about what has captured your imagination.

Years ago, long before I was a writer, I was struck by an article in a health magazine. I yanked it out and noticed the writer's name. A few years later, writing became more interesting to me as a career possibility. I kept seeing that writer's byline and learned that she lived about 45 minutes from me. On a whim, I searched her out on the internet, found an email address, and sent her an invitation to lunch. To my surprise, she said yes. Years later, Melba Newsome remains one of my professional mentors and has become a dear friend. My first conversations with her gave me enough information to know how to put my career in place, and our ensuing conversations over the years have been a delightful gift. Granted, talking to someone once doesn't replace immersing yourself in learning about the subject, but it can often give you enough insight to begin.

What does plugging into our dreams have to do with self-image and body image? It is in realizing our dreams that we access our truest happiness; and when we are happy, we feel better about ourselves.

Today ⟶ Is there someone you know who can help you go further on your journey? If so, reach out to him or her and see what comes from the effort.

— 218 —

Give For a Minute

Two of my favorite websites are www.goodsearch.com and www.greater good.com. With each one, I can do something daily that is bigger than me and allows me to support efforts that I believe in. At GoodSearch, I do searches just like I would on Google. For each search, the nonprofit of my choice is given a penny. As much as I search each day, that adds up to a lot of pennies for Circle de Luz (my nonprofit of choice). At GreaterGood, you are introduced to a network of websites that support great causes at no cost to you. All you have to do is click through to a site associated with a cause that's important to you. For each click (limit one per day per site) sponsors pay a royalty to the nonprofit, leading to significant funding for things like mammography programs, ending world hunger, or preserving rain forests.

Today ——⟶ Go to www.goodsearch.com and www.greatergood.com and contribute to these meaningful causes. By responding to the world's needs, you widen your circle of concern and influence.

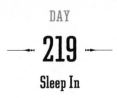

— 219 —

Sleep In

Been incredibly busy lately? Well, when *isn't* that the case? We run ourselves so ragged at times that we often forget to stop and meet our basic needs.

Today —— Sleep in. Turn off the alarm clock and wake up naturally.

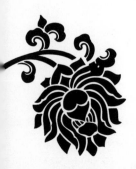

— 220 —

Be There

For several summers, I worked at a teen enrichment program. Before each summer's program kicked off, the staff went away for a retreat. The very first rule that the retreat facilitator would write on his flip chart was always "If You Are Here, Be Here." Life is at its most pure when we are mentally present in just one place at a time. When we can fully engage with where we are, our best self shows up.

Polly Campbell, the spirituality writer, recommends just trying to be mindful in the second. If you do find your mind wandering, don't berate yourself, just remind yourself to refocus.

For example, let's say your mind wanders during your child's school conference. Begin by asking the teacher if she can repeat what she said. Then, Campbell says, "Pay attention. Clue in to the teacher at that moment by using your senses. Realize what the chair feels like, what her face looks like."

Later, she recommends, go back and think about why your mind was tempted to wander. "Ask yourself, 'What was that? Is there something that I don't want to deal with or am I overwhelmed?'"

Today —— Practice mindfulness and be there in every place that you are.

— 221 —

Learn Something from Your Mom

There are infinite things I have learned from my mom, not the least of which is that Murphy Oil Soap will get any stain out, including cooking oil. The things I've learned from my mom have made me a more competent woman, but there is still so much more she can teach me: the secret to her fabulous hash brown potatoes, how she gets plants to take root in South Carolina's unfertile soil and blazing sun, and her secrets to mending clothing mishaps by hand, to name just a few. By engaging with our mothers through their talents, we allow ourselves to see them as whole women not just in the singular category of "our mom." We also allow ourselves to grow as women.

Today — If she is still alive, learn something from your mom. Maybe it's how she prunes the roses in her yard or the trick to her fabulous soufflé. Maybe you want her to teach you the art of book preservation or how to fix a dropped stitch. Whatever it is that your mom does well, ask her to share it with you today (if she lives far away, you can still learn things from your mom over the phone). Cherish what you learn from and about her.

— 222 —

Nurture Something

Irecently had dinner with a friend who relayed a conversation she'd had with her doctor about a year ago, after anxiety and panic drove her to make an appointment. She thought she was in danger of having a heart attack. Her doctor took her vitals, asked probing questions, and ultimately told her that her problem wasn't physiological, it was psychological. She needed to pursue some hobbies, he said, and she needed to get a tomato plant. A year later it turns out her doctor's orders were just right.

"Do you have a tomato plant?" I asked.

"I have about seven plants now," she answered, with a smile that revealed how much better she was doing now than she was a year ago. My friend wasn't better just because of the tomato plant, but the tomato plant itself symbolized so much: her ability to take her happiness into her own hands, her ability to nurture and sustain her vitality.

Today —— Choose something to grow and nurture. Maybe it's a violet plant that reminds you of your mom, or an orchid plant because you love the way they look. Whatever you choose, make sure it is something that will bring you joy over time. If it doesn't come with a container, choose one you like, pick up some potting soil, and get started.

— 223 —

Listen to Your Body and Respond

We spend a whole lot of time berating our bodies and not nearly enough time caring for them. It's time to start focusing on being responsive to our body's needs.

Today — Every hour today (set an alarm if you need to remind yourself) stop and ask yourself, "What am I feeling right now? What do I need?" The idea is to give your mind and body what it needs—sustenance, fluids, a stretch, a time out, a laugh, a diversion—whenever it needs it, rather than running around for hours and realizing you have yet to meet a need that will help your body operate better.

Write Thank-You Notes

In this age of emailing and texting, I have fallen in love with handwritten thank-you notes. I just love to send them. The stationery I choose delights me, writing the note humbles me and roots me in my gratitude. After the note is sealed and addressed, I feel so much goodwill that the note, I find, is much more for me than it is for the person to whom it is addressed. When I write thank-you notes, I am reminded that my life is blessed and that wellspring of gratitude is restorative.

Today —— If you don't have any lovely stationery, pick some up and then sit for a bit and write thank-you notes for recent kindnesses that have come your way. Revel in the blessings that have been given to you and the lovely relationships that have allowed them to happen.

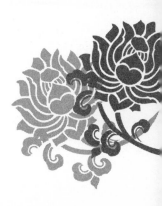

— 225 —

Learn about the Middle Way

If there is anything absolute about my personality, it is that I am generally even-keeled. If you were to ask the college or high school students I've taught over the years to recall a time that I got mad, I think only about three instances would come up—and those incidents were set off because someone entered my no-fly zone by acting intolerant or disrespectful, or taking advantage of someone else.

The thing about being even-keeled is that there aren't a lot of highs, but there are also very few, if any, lows. Nothing seems impossible or upending to me, nor does anything feel like my own private Oscar's night. It's all just life, lived one day at a time.

When I was an undergraduate, I took a course on Buddhism and I felt such a connection with many of its teachings. The one that seemed the most familiar to me, then and now, is the concept of the "Middle Way" or "Middle Path."

Put generally, the Middle Way is the Buddhist practice of nonextremism. It is the path of moderation, where you stay away from the extremes of sensual indulgence and austerity. Instead, you aim for something in between, and try to maintain a practice of wisdom, morality, and observation.

As spirituality writer Polly Campbell says, "When you are centered in spirit, you are able to see your purpose more clearly. You are able to solve problems more effectively because you are open to the information coming to you. It allows you to see a more whole picture of your life. When you can do that, you are going to live it more wholly."

The gift of the Middle Way is that it invites a balanced approach to life, a belief that nothing is too urgent or dire. Take it a step further and you realize that our appearance simply exists, it is neither good nor bad.

Today ⟶ Take some time to learn about the concept of the Middle Way by researching it on the Internet or checking out a book. Consider how you can adopt some of its philosophy in your quest toward a more autonomous self.

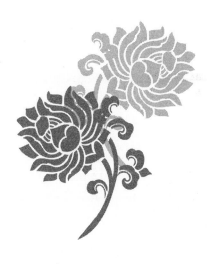

— 226 —

Revel in Your Accomplishments

I don't just have a to-do list. I have a to-do notebook, with lists broken down by what I will do each day. Every Friday, I plan the next week, considering exactly what I want to accomplish each day. Most days, I knock out no more than half of what's on my list. With those sorts of odds, it would be easy to feel unsuccessful. And feeling unsuccessful is just an opening to feeling inadequate in other ways. Unfortunately, discouragement can be a slippery slope.

Today —— Revel in your accomplishments. Open your *Beautiful You* journal and write down everything that you have accomplished in the last week. Recognizing just how much you are accomplishing is a wonderful reminder of your abilities and energy. So instead of seeing what I *don't* do at the end of each day, I focus on what I did. I use a highlighter to mark off each accomplishment, so those items jump off the page at me at the end of the day instead of the items left undone.

DAY

— 227 —

Create a Bedtime Ritual

Going to bed was always a race for me. How quickly could I brush my teeth, take out my contacts, and change clothes before getting into bed? But I have learned that the rush of getting to bed didn't calm me, it jacked me up.

By creating a bedtime ritual where I wash my face, put on moisturizer, brush and floss my teeth, update my journal, and read a few pages of my book, I provide myself quiet time to unwind, to reflect on the day that just ended, and to think about the day that is coming. It's not that my bedtime ritual makes me more physically beautiful, it's that it provides me with the opportunity to be deliberately still and thoughtful at the end of the day.

Today — Create a three- to five-step bedtime ritual that will allow you to unwind, savor, reflect, and plan before going to sleep.

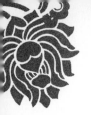

Say Yes

In "Beyond Stereotypes: Rebuilding the Foundation of Beauty Beliefs," a 2005 study commissioned by the beauty-product brand Dove, two-thirds of women and girls revealed that they avoid activities such as meeting friends, voicing an opinion, going to school, going to work, exercising, dating, or even seeking medical care because they don't like the way they look. Have you ever skipped an event because you weren't comfortable with how you looked? What did missing that event or experience add to your life? What would going have added to your life?

Today ⎯⎯ Say yes to the things that you would normally skip because of your displeasure with your appearance. Your body doesn't experience your life—your soul does. When you deny yourself a pleasurable experience, you are punishing your soul.

See a Nutritionist

I f food has occupied an unhealthy place in your mind or life, it is difficult to assume a normal relationship with it just because a book tells you to do so. One way to establish a healthier relationship with food is to visit with a nutritionist for some education.

Today —⁓ Think your relationship with food has been unhealthy? Schedule an appointment to visit a nutritionist. Your local hospital or physician can make a recommendation and some insurance plans will cover the visit. Let the nutrition expert know you want to learn about healthy eating and how you can best fuel your body. Take good notes so you can move forward with new insight.

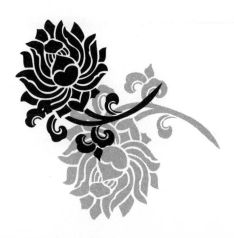

Shift Your Outlook

How we live our lives is greatly influenced by our perceptions. A change in point of view can broaden our perspective. When we enhance our outlook, things shimmer in a different way. We realize how conditioned our viewpoint is and can begin to open to change.

Today —— Do something that alters a perception you have of yourself. Wear something that is *so* not you. Sit with someone different at a meeting or at lunch, or take a different seat in the classroom. Take a class at the gym that you have never taken before. Do something that shakes things up for you and then consider how that one simple change altered the way you looked at things today.

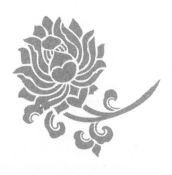

— 231 —

Consider What You Need

So much of our self-doubt comes from believing that we are not adequately prepared for what we might be facing. We lose sight of the fact that we are fully equipped to become better prepared. Do you need to learn more about a certain subject? Then check out a book, call an expert, or surf the web. Realize that you have more power than you imagined and you can operate from a place of strength rather than fear.

Today —— Ask yourself this question in your *Beautiful You* Journal: What can I do to prepare for what I am facing? After reviewing your answer, act on your observation.

DAY

— 232 —

Find Your True Comfort Ritual

I was twenty-three, fresh out of college, and in my first year of teaching when my college boyfriend and I broke up. It was an amicable break-up; I knew we would continue to be the best of friends. The afternoon of our break-up, I had just stopped my tears when I came across a note he had left for me; it was inside a book of his that I had wanted to read. The sweetness of it, the pain of it, the honesty of it undid me. In the living room of the apartment I shared with another teacher, who was a dear friend, I collapsed back into tears. Heather had never seen me cry, and after listening to me and letting me cry for a bit, she pulled me off the couch and took me to get my very first manicure. It seems a small gesture, but I remember it as a valuable lesson Heather taught me. We have it within our power to get up again, and we also have it within our power to bring ourselves comfort.

I often hear people talk about how food is their friend, how it provides them comfort when nothing else will. The truth is that food doesn't really provide all that much comfort. It can be soothing in the moment, like chicken noodle soup when you are sick, but food—or anything else we binge on—rarely makes us feel better overall. It simply makes us feel better in that moment. Afterwards, we feel worse for allowing ourselves to finish a whole bag, box, or gallon of whatever it was we used to get our fix.

If we can find something that really comforts us, we will be able to take care of our true need without creating a new need—the desire to assuage the guilt we feel over a food binge.

Today ⟶ Consider what really brings you comfort when you are experiencing an emotion that needs an outlet. Is it journaling, taking a nap, lighting a candle, enjoying a massage, reading, taking a bubble bath, getting a pedicure, confiding in a friend, going for a run? Give yourself that gift the next time you need comfort and savor the fact that you can give yourself the care you need.

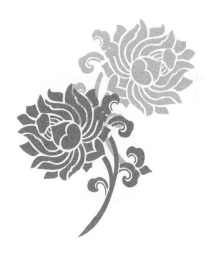

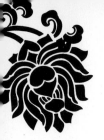

— 233 —

Make a Meal from Scratch

Our lives can get so busy that we see meals as a nuisance, something to quickly sneak in so we can keep going. Or we get so obsessive about food that we see it is an enemy, something that teases us away from what we want for ourselves. We can give food too much power. Sometimes, we just need to accept the fact that it is our fuel and be grateful that we can have a hand in nurturing ourselves by preparing foods that fuel us.

Today —— Make a meal from scratch.

— 234 —

Touch

There is a reason why an infant stops crying when you pick her up. That simple touch calms her nervous system and makes her feel better immediately. Touch is an amazing thing. I always enjoyed a good back rub or holding hands, but it wasn't until we began to research adoption that I really came to understand how touch boosts one's entire sympathetic system by building neurons and developing synapses.

"Hold him all the time," our pediatrician told us as we prepared to pick up our son. The deep, gentle pressure of being held is soothing input for an infant. Touch, it turns out, is a natural healing remedy that we often overlook, something that increases our sense of well-being with almost no effort.

Today ⸻ Hold someone's hand or rub a back. Enjoy the sensation for more than just a fleeting moment. Bask in the wash of good feelings you receive from that interaction.

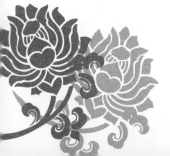

— 235 —

Set Limits

I was painfully thin in high school. It wasn't that I had a desire to be thin. It was that I had a desire to be busy, to be doing, to be going, and food—specifically, slowing down for meals—simply got in the way of that. I existed on a pack of plain M&Ms and seemingly endless cans of Pepsi each day. Not only was I thin, I was likely malnourished.

Fast forward to my mid-twenties, when regular meals became a part of my life. I filled out, reaching a normal weight for my size. But when someone is used to seeing you one way, that person may be surprised or worried when you fill out. I can't say for sure what motivated her, but my mamacita, who is a good woman and meant absolutely no harm, often had my weight on her mind. When we talked on the phone, she often brought it up, encouraging me to get back to my high school weight, a weight that I knew was dangerously low. I'd hang up with her feeling hurt and frustrated.

One day, I finally decided that talking about my body was off limits and that I needed to let her know that. If I didn't tell my mom that talk about my weight was harming our relationship, making me want to talk to her less, then I was denying her the opportunity to care for me, as well as the opportunity to change. She is a sweet, well-meaning woman who was simply projecting onto me her greatest fear for herself, so she deserved to know that she was hurting me. The next time she made a weight comment, I stopped her. "Mom, we need to get off the phone now. I'm not mad at you, but this is not an appropriate conversation and I don't want to frustrate either of us by going on with it," I told her.

She sputtered for a moment, surprised. She pleaded for a moment, but I held firm and said, before hanging up, "I'll talk to you in a few days. I love you." I sat in the bedroom of my apartment, looking around at the trappings of my adult life, my stomach gurgling a bit with worry. Had I hurt her? Would she be mad? Should I call her back? And then I stopped myself, because I knew that what I had done in that moment was to teach both my mother and me that I could rescue myself.

It took a few more times for that firm reminder to create a new pattern in our phone calls. But more than ten years later, my weight—whether it's a little up or a little down—remains off limits with my mother. In the end, she didn't care so much about my weight; she cared about my happiness. She knows that I am healthy, that I eat well and work out, and she accepts that who I am now is simply who I am, not someone who needs tweaking to get back to her seventeen-year-old self.

Today —— If there is a recurring conversation in your life that hurts you, realize that it is okay to set limits by letting someone know that he or she is hurting you and that you will not accept it. This might mean you have to tell someone you love (and who you know loves you back) to bite her tongue rather than continue to offer her unsolicited or impolite feedback to you. You are also teaching yourself that you can protect yourself from unwitting attacks on your self-esteem.

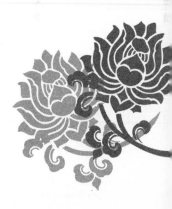

— 236 —

Accentuate the Positive

B ecoming more positive and optimistic about ourselves and our situations simply takes practice. By deliberately being more positive than negative, we develop that general outlook. And when we feel more positive about ourselves, we are clearing the way to recognizing our own brilliance.

Today —— In your *Beautiful You* journal, consider what feels good about where you are right now. Why does it feel like you are on the right track? What are the benefits of this part of your journey? By reminding ourselves of the upside of our current situation, we recognize both the control we have and the possibility before us.

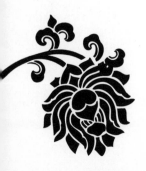

Do a Little Searching

I am a sucker for any quiz. I love doing a little private investigation into myself, and a little private investigation can lead to a whole lot of self-knowledge. Needless to say, when I came across the Self-Directed Search, a career inventory that you can take online for $9.95, I had to do it. And here's what the thirty-minute test revealed about me: I am inclined toward a career that is social, artistic, and enterprising (with "investigative" a close fourth) and should stay away from careers that involve the mechanical and technological. No surprise there. It also suggested careers for me, some of which I have already tackled in some way: teacher, community organization director, editor, and columnist or commentator. But the inventory also had a few career suggestions that surprised me: minister/priest/rabbi, food and drug inspector, arbitrator, cosmetologist, choreographer, comedian, magician, sign shop supervisor, and paper goods production supervisor.

The list helped me assess how much of a handle I had on my strengths and whether or not I was using those strengths in what I do professionally. When we're aligned with our strengths, we're able to move more confidently in the world.

Today —— Visit www.self-directed-search.com and complete the career inventory. When you receive your results, open up your *Beautiful You* journal and write them down. Consider what the list reveals about you. How are you using the strengths and talents identified by the career inventory? How can you use them in a more effective way?

— 238 —

Visualize

Whenever I am giving a new talk or workshop, I prepare as much as I possibly can. But I inevitably feel a rush of anxiety as the event approaches. The final part of my preparation is to visualize the workshop. Even if it is just for a minute, I see myself in the presentation space, imagine the audience there, and move through different parts of the program. That visualization always seems to calm me and gives me a sense of confidence. Later, when I stand before my audience, I can access that calm again because it feels like I've done it before.

Today —— Visualize yourself successfully doing something that would usually give you anxiety. Now notice and enjoy the calm and confidence brought on by that exercise.

— 239 —

Learn as Much as You Can

Confidence comes from a certainty that we have the skills and sensitivities to handle what comes before us. A student who walks confidently into an exam is the one who knows she has studied and retained the information she has been taught. The insecure student knows she has not learned what she is being asked to demonstrate. Knowledge, it seems, is a critical part of confidence—whether it is knowledge that will be tested on an exam or the kind that helps us manage our responsibilities. The more you know, the better prepared you feel to handle what's before you. And the better prepared you feel, the more confident you are.

Today — Consider the subjects that are incredibly interesting to you and choose one on which to become an expert. Perhaps it is creativity or body image or philanthropy or education or true crime or adoption or youth gangs or ethnicity and race or football. (Oh wait, those are the subjects *I* am terribly interested in!) Whatever your interests, choose one and bury yourself in it to gain a better understanding. Pick up a book on the subject and crack it open. Do a web search or set Google Alerts to automatically send you news articles about the subject. Begin filling your mind with information and you'll feel your confidence soar.

DAY

— 240 —

Watch a Movie that Speaks of Empowerment

We all have movies that just make us want to applaud because of their "kick some ass" messages. For me, it's *Real Women Have Curves*. There's no boy of relevance to speak of; it's just a girl in a fight that will define her life— a fight for education, a fight against being critiqued by a beauty standard that was not created with her in mind.

Come to think of it, I have more than one favorite empowerment movie. *Erin Brockovich, Bend It Like Beckham, Akeelah and the Bee,* and *Little Miss Sunshine* all make me feel pretty pumped, and they are just the sort of fare I turn to when I wish to be reminded of my power and possibility.

Today — Watch a movie that inspires you with its message of empowerment. A quick poll on my blog lead readers to suggest *Sisterhood of the Traveling Pants, Little Women, Hairspray, Girlfight, Freedom Writers, Charlie's Angels, Baby Boom, Chocolat, Norma Rae, Nine to Five, Alien, Pretty in Pink, In the Time of the Butterflies, The Joy Luck Club, Iron Jawed Angels, Bordertown,* and *Terminator 2* as some options.

— 241 —

Take a Cooking Class

A nother way to enhance your relationship with food and turn eating into a more intentional experience is to take a cooking class.

Today —— Sign up for a cooking class that features healthy cuisine. Try your local gourmet grocer or a college's continuing education program for some options.

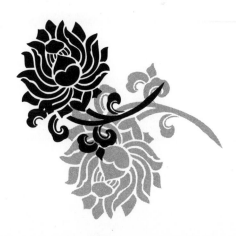

— 242 —

Say I Love You

Do you remember the exact moment that someone said "I love you"? It doesn't have to be a romantic moment; maybe a parent, a friend, or a sibling said it to you. Chances are there is at least one "I love you" seared into your memory; likely, there are several more. Why do we remember "I love you" moments when there is so much more we forget over time? It's because the words "I love you" let us know that someone else values us, that our worth is recognized and embraced, that we are compelling. We cherish statements of love we have received, but we don't always remember to give them out as much as we should.

Today ——➤ Tell the people you love that you love them. Say "I love you" deliberately and enjoy both the warmth it gives you and the boost of confidence it is likely to give them.

— 243 —

Realize That Some Days Are Just Hard

One December morning, I woke with a sinus infection and a raging rosacea flare-up. My cheeks and nose were so swollen, I didn't look like myself. Meanwhile, I had gone to sleep the night before immediately after my shower and my curly hair had dried in a way that, well, inspired thoughts of Sideshow Bob from *The Simpsons*. The reflection that looked back at me from the mirror was not one I was thrilled with, and yet there wasn't anything I could do about it.

I didn't have time to take a new shower because my baby boy was up and ready for my full attention. The cream I had for my rosacea wasn't working. I couldn't go to the doctor to treat my puffy-face-inducing sinus infection because there was no one to watch my boy. I was just going to have to deal, which would have been easier if I were just planning to hang out all day, but I was hosting a party for more than fifty people that night. For a minute, I started worrying about how I would look. But then I got over it because the party I was hosting was going to raise money for various cash-strapped nonprofits in our area. People weren't coming to see my skin or hair. They weren't going to care what I looked like. For me to enjoy the night, I needed to not care too.

Today —— Realize that no matter how much you try to beat the self-defeating racket in your head, some days will still be hard. You won't like what you see in the mirror because it's not what you are used to or what you have come to expect. And that's fine. It doesn't mean that you are any less worthy of love and respect that day. It just serves to remind you that you always have a choice; you can always say no to the racket, and in doing so, you're saying yes to yourself.

DAY

— 244 —

Get Photographed

Iloathe being photographed, but I've learned that professional photographers know how to wrestle your photographic demons. The professionals can bring out your true self in photographs; you won't see your flaws and imperfections, you'll see what everyone else sees, which is pretty darn fabulous.

I met a photographer once who was doing a series of nudes, shooting women of all ages and backgrounds in preparation for an exhibit. She needed women of color and older women for her exhibit, so I sent some of my friends her way. Those friends told me later that the resulting photographs, in which they were stripped of the exterior trappings they thought made them unique, actually captured their true spirits. Many professional photographers, however, are skilled at bringing forth the essence of their subjects whether or not they are nude.

Today — Sign up for a session with a professional photographer (and it doesn't have to be in the nude). By having a professional capture your true essence, you will have a record to remind you every day of your radiance and beauty.

Speak Up

We all want to feel valued and appreciated, and we get that in a variety of ways, including from our many accomplishments. When we engage in the world, we see our ideas, our abilities, our care, and our concern enhance it—through the classes we participate in or teach, the work we do, the efforts we support, the sports we play, the groups we belong to, the relationships we have with our friends, family, or partner, and the pets we nurture, among other things. It is unfortunate that sometimes our lack of confidence keeps us from really engaging in the world, denying us the opportunity to feel connected and thus valued and appreciated.

Today —— Speak up. Share your ideas or experiences and see how much value you add to the world.

— 246 —

Create an Inspiration Board

As a college sophomore, I knew what I wanted for myself, but some-times I would forget it and focus instead on whatever was immediately in front of me. The trouble was, the things that were immediately in front of me didn't always move me forward in my life. So that summer, I decided to create a visual representation of what I envisioned for myself. With poster board, tape, scissors, and a stack of magazines, I created a collage. The collage hung on my wall for the next two years, a daily reminder of who I wished to become and how I wished to get there. It was a moment where I knew I was taking my life into my own hands, choosing to make things happen rather than allowing things to happen to me. That sort of self-empowerment always boosts a person's self-esteem. Though it was inspired by wishful thinking, it truly became my willful thinking.

Today —— Gather your supplies—a bulletin board or poster board, magazines and photos, tape, and scissors—and create your own inspiration board. Use images and words that speak to you and show what you imagine for yourself. When you're done, write the date on the back and place it somewhere you'll come across it regularly. Becoming empowered and self-possessed starts with a vision.

DAY

— 247 —

Thank Your Body

We spend so much time harping on what our bodies *can't* do, on how they *don't* look, that we forget to celebrate what our bodies do for us every day. Today we are expressing gratitude for our bodies. Not only will it reframe our focus, it will also boost our happiness.

Today —— In your *Beautiful You* journal, write a thank-you letter to your body. In what ways does it support you, do more than you ask, or even pleasantly surprise you? Appreciate all that it makes possible.

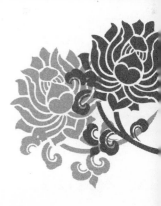

— 248 —

Watch Your Children's Language

One fall morning, my nephew told my sister that he couldn't wear his karate uniform because only girls wore them.

"Why does he think that?" I asked my sister.

"Hmmm. There are ten kids in his class and only two of them are girls. Both the boys and the girls had their uniforms on so I don't know why he thinks that," she answered.

My sister was terribly aware that her three-year-old son was already forming limiting thoughts about gender. That realization put her on alert.

Children tell us so much with their language. It is important for us to listen to what they are saying and respond appropriately so that negative messages about beauty, body, and gender are not further perpetuated over generations and time.

Today —— Watch your children's language. What are they saying that you need to respond to and address?

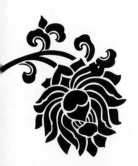

—•— 249 —•—

Consult a Make-Up Artist

While I don't think women need to wear makeup every day or even at all, makeup can be a fun way to express ourselves and highlight our features. But just because you are female doesn't mean you inherently know what types of products or shades are right for you, or even how to use them. Consulting a professional can make you feel more confident about creating the look you wish to create while properly caring for your skin.

Today —— Visit a department store make-up counter or a cosmetics store and find someone whose look is one you might wish to emulate or whose approach makes you feel comfortable. Tell her what you want and what you are struggling with. Ask plenty of questions while she puts together a look for you. If possible, watch the process with a handheld mirror so that you get a visual lesson as well.

— 250 —

Get in Touch

I have a close friend in Ohio who I used to teach with in my early to mid-twenties. We were kindred souls from the moment we met and have never run out of things to say to each other. Being with her—heck, just talking to her—does my heart good, but I have this funny way of not giving myself permission to call her as often as I'd like. It seems that every time I get on the road to Charlotte, a drive that takes me about twenty-five to thirty minutes, I think of calling her, but then I don't because I think "thirty minutes isn't enough time" or "this probably isn't a good time for her." Instead, I put off the phone call, waiting for when we can talk for at least an hour... but of course the hour never comes. When we do finally get a hold of each other, it's pure joy, even if we can only talk for twenty minutes.

This year, I finally had a little chat with myself and said, "You no longer have side-by-side classrooms or the same planning period, so it is always going to be impossible to catch up one hundred percent. Enjoying each other a little today is more than a gracious plenty." And sure enough, every conversation with her has been more than just a gracious plenty—it's been a sustaining plenty, too; fuel for my life until we can talk again.

Today —— Call someone you adore but haven't talked to in a while because you were avoiding all the catch up. Don't worry about bringing him or her up to speed on everything, just enjoy the conversation.

— 251 —

Consider Your Journey

As you know, sitting down to write in your journal is a way of nurturing yourself. Reflection helps you to grow, nudges you a step closer to your brilliance as you reflect and interpret what has passed before you. Journaling allows you to see what seems familiar in new ways.

Today —— In your *Beautiful You* journal, answer these questions: What were you doing at this time last year? What has changed? What has stayed the same?

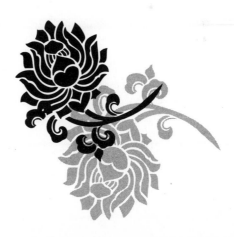

— 252 —

Vote with Your Dollar

We have talked already about how in order for the media to change, we have to resist its inappropriate messages. Once you quit accepting society's standards of beauty and clear your mind of that verbal and visual clutter, you can make room for what *you* think and feel is beautiful. Eventually, if enough of us do it, we change the media.

Earlier this year, you examined the magazines and television shows you were watching. Now, to change the nature of marketing, we have to resist buying into the bag of goods we are being sold. If we buy products from companies whose ads use fear, stereotypes, or manipulation, to appeal to us, we are sending marketers messages and giving them positive reinforcement.

Today —— Don't buy the hype. Consider a product's media campaign before making a purchase. Even if you really are excited about what the product promises to deliver, consider the messages sent by its marketing campaign before you buy it. If it's negative—if it sexualizes or demoralizes or demeans or endangers women or girls, or if it does anything else that is questionable—skip it. There is another product available to you that will do the same thing; buy that one. Or consider going without it completely. When we resist the message, we deliver a message.

Want to amplify the volume of your message? Send a letter to the company telling them that you are opting out on their product because of their marketing techniques.

DAY

— 253 —

Say Prayers Rooted in Strength and Gratitude

As a person of faith, I have found two prayers that most sustain me. Because I believe that I am ultimately responsible for making the best possible decisions; because I believe that I have what I need to make those decisions and will be given anything else I might need; because I believe that if I have no control over the outcome of a situation, then that actually means that what happened was likely meant to be—for a reason that may only be made clear to me later or never—I focus my prayers on requesting strength or offering thanks.

Faced with a difficult situation, I pray for the wisdom or grace to handle the situation well. Faced with good fortune, I offer my thanks for the gifts that I have been given. When my loved ones or the world face difficult challenges, I ask that we may be given the guidance, resolve, clarity, and sensitivity needed to deal with those situations. When good fortune smiles down, I smile upward. Both prayers ground me and give me exactly what I need; they root me to my truest self and to the universe.

I don't offer these prayers at a certain time or on a particular schedule; in many ways, that makes it easier for me to offer them. Perhaps that is because I avoid the strict rules about prayer that some of us faced in our childhood. As writer Polly Campbell explains, "Most of us were raised to believe that there were rules to prayer." When there are rules, we can become resistant. By offering my prayers whenever the notion flashes into my mind, I am always in touch with something bigger than myself, and that's infinitely helpful.

Campbell also suggests that prayer seems to improve the quality of one's life. With prayer, she says, "The universe opens up to you in a way that has your highest purpose in mind."

Today —— Even if you don't consider yourself a religious or spiritual person, try to act from a place of faith by considering what prayers for strength or of thanks you might offer to the God of your understanding or to the universe. Then, in a quiet moment, offer them. Those prayers take absolutely nothing away from you, and they could add calm, hope, clarity, or a sense of purpose to your day.

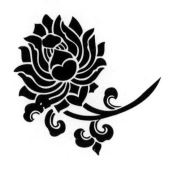

— 254 —

Send Birthday Cards

Celebrating the people in our lives in an intentional way helps to build our gratitude. When we take the time to appreciate others, we nurture our connections, build our relationships, and reflect on the joy people have brought into our lives. By practicing gratitude and reflection, we build confidence and increase feelings of well-being.

One simple way to celebrate the people in our lives is by acknowledging their birthdays, if even in a simple way.

Today —— Create a birthday calendar, a month-by-month list of birthdays you want to remember. Or use the birthday reminders feature at www.alerts. com. Next, go ahead and pick up birthday cards for this month's and next month's birthday girls and boys, and take the time to write a short note in each card. If you don't have time to hit the local card shop, try www.jack cards.com: you can select cards online and they will be mailed to you when it's time to mail them to your loved ones.

As for notes, I like to start each birthday greeting I send with the words "I celebrate your..." and then I fill in the blank for each loved one. After all, who doesn't want to know what you love about them? When you mail that card, you make yourself and someone else feel good.

— 255 —

Encourage a Healthy but Relaxed Attitude about Food

So often, the root cause of our food anxieties is really someone else's food anxiety: the mom who always maligned food, the dad who commented on what you were eating, the girlfriend who kept saying, "Oh, I can't" to one type of food or another. By vilifying food, we create not just fear but obsession—in ourselves and in those who watch us. And obsession forces us to lose both our connection to our centers and our ability to lead ourselves from a place of intentionality.

Today — Regardless of whether or not you have children, set a good example for the children in your life by eating the food you'd like them to eat, and show them that treats can be enjoyed if our approach to them is sensible. Don't worry so much about talking the talk. Today, just walk the walk and have a healthy, relaxed, appropriate attitude toward food.

— 256 —

Dress Fresh

When I was both a high school and college student, I would always dress up on a test or exam day. Normally a jeans and T-shirt, rugby shirt, or oxford-shirt girl, dressing up gave me a different air on those days when I wanted to be my most focused. For whatever reason, changing it up for my exams usually worked. (Well, except in calculus. Nothing—not tutors, attending office hours, or dressing up—worked for calculus). Just sitting up a little bit straighter as I worked gave me more confidence, and that confidence improved my performance.

Today, I have taken a step back even from the jeans and oxfords. I'm a yoga pants and hoodie girl. But I find that every time I change it up a little, even with jeans and a blouse, I feel more confident and capable. The way I portray myself changes the way I perceive myself, and sometimes feeling like a competent professional is exactly what I need.

Today —— Look past the old staples in your closet when you get dressed this morning and dress fresh. Giving yourself a fresh look for the day will likely translate into a fresh outlook.

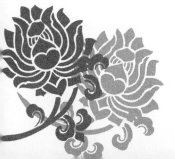

— 257 —

Make Dinner for Someone Else

One of my favorite things to do is to make a meal for a friend or loved one I know can use a break. I know it is helpful to my loved one, but preparing that meal, being able to express my care for someone else, is helpful to me as well. Sometimes one of the most nurturing things we can do for ourselves is nurture someone else. It reminds us of our truest heart, allows us to realize our best intentions, and boosts our understanding of ourselves.

Today —— Cook a meal for yourself tonight that allows you to also create a portion for someone else. Package it in a container that doesn't need to be returned to you and include heating instructions. Then deliver it to that person you've been thinking about and enjoy the smile it puts on her face and yours.

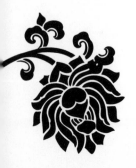

— 258 —

Watch Wildlife

The beauty of Discovery Channel's *Planet Earth* documentary series almost moved me to tears. As I watched episode after episode, I couldn't help but feel like the world was so big and I was so small. Sometimes, a reminder of the vastness of our world is just what we need to help us realize that our insecurities are insignificant.

Today —— Tune into a wildlife show on the Discovery Channel or Animal Planet. Don't have cable? Rent a series like *Plant Earth* or a movie like *March of the Penguins*. While you learn about the eating habits of the great white shark or the nesting habits of leatherback turtles, you'll be led away from your myopic view of life. Taking yourself as far away as possible from the world of beauty standards and self-critique broadens your views and gives you new perspective.

— 259 —

Get to Know Your Breasts

B reast self-exams are now considered more optional than mandatory, but I still know more than a handful of women who found their breast cancer themselves, and plenty of doctors still consider them an important part of the early detection process.

Dr. Laura Danile of Charlotte Radiology in Charlotte, North Carolina had this to say on the topic: "The concept of breast self-exams has fallen under scrutiny because current medical literature does not show evidence that it improves breast cancer mortality rates. While it is difficult to dispute the available published data, I still believe there is definite value in the performance of the breast self-exam. On one level, it allows a woman to become familiar with how her normal breast tissue feels so that she might be able to detect a change which could signify cancer. More than that, though, it promotes women taking an active and, hopefully, proactive role in their health maintenance. The greatest source of empowerment is being in control of yourself and taking responsibility for the betterment of your life."

Today —— Open your calendar and schedule a monthly appointment with yourself for a complete breast self-exam. You might do a skin examination on the same day. For more information on self-exams, visit www.nationalbreast-cancer.org/about-breast-cancer/Breast-Self-Exam.aspx.

— 260 —

Pay Off Debt

Debt. Too often we accrue it because we want to look good and feel good, and we're convinced that the only way we can do that is by spending a significant amount of money—money we don't have in cash at the moment. The truth is that you don't need to spend a lot of money to be your best. Only when we separate ourselves from thinking about what money can do for us do we begin to understand what we can do for ourselves.

Today ——— You've already made a budget. Now take it a step further by making a master list of how much you owe and to whom. Create a plan that will allow you to actively pay off your debt while not accruing more. Need help? Check out the library for some great books on women and money, such as *The Money Therapist*, by Marcia Brixey.

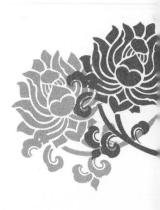

Laugh

When two girlfriends came to town, I took them out to dinner at a nice Mexican restaurant I was eager to share with them.

"Make sure to listen to the specials," I told them. "They're always really good."

The waiter, one I knew because I had been enjoying that restaurant's carne asada and sabana de res for years, stopped by our table and very ceremoniously began sharing the specials with us in that trademark formal waiter voice.

"We have grilled kangaroo with mole sauce."

Hold the friggin' phone! I thought. There was no way I heard that right. We were in a Mexican restaurant in small town North Carolina!

"Did you say *kangaroo?*" I asked, incredulous.

"Kangaroo," he said, nodding, and then kept going without missing a beat.

Okay, clearly I wasn't hearing things right, but I knew my friends had heard what I asked and I knew that any minute they would be bent over laughing. What I heard couldn't have been what he'd said, I thought. *Did he say carne a jus, maybe?* I was trying to figure it out while he continued explaining the specials. Then, suddenly I was overcome. I felt a laugh coming up from my belly. *Must. Not. Laugh. In. This. Fine. Restaurant.* But it came out anyway, clearly a laugh, so I feigned a cough and said excuse me.

One of my friend's eyes darted toward me. Don't look at me, I thought, and I turned my face toward the wall, drawing out my faux coughing fit. When he had made his way back to the kitchen, all three of us burst out laughing: me at the fact that I clearly hadn't heard him right; them at the fact that I was busted for bad behavior at the table. No, you heard it right, they assured me. He said kangaroo.

The rest of the weekend, we passed Kangaroo gas stations left and right—it was a company I never even noticed existed before that weekend—and we would melt into fits of giggles again. Even now, remembering the story, I am laughing.

Laughter is so joyful. It makes you feel so alive, so present, so invested in something. Laughter—cliché be damned—is indeed good medicine.

Today ⟶ Laugh. Visit an online site like www.jokes.com or www.jibjab .com, watch a comedy that always guarantees you'll laugh, or see the humor in something your friend, partner, or coworker says—just let yourself indulge in a good, true laugh. Laughter raises endorphin levels, relieves stress, makes you feel more cheerful, invigorates the mind, and stimulates the immune system—all things that bring out your brilliance.

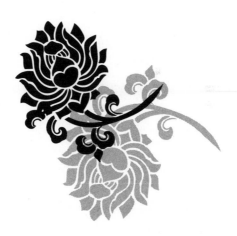

— 262 —

Think About Your Vitality

Laughter, indeed, makes you feel vital and alive, but it's not the only thing that can make you feel that way.

Today —— In your *Beautiful You* journal, answer these questions. When have you felt most alive? Why was that?

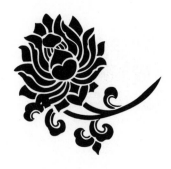

— 263 —

Watch *Absolutely Safe*

*A*bsolutely Safe, a documentary by Carol Ciancutti-Leyva, looks at the controversy over breast-implant safety. I watch this film with my body image class every semester, and while there are moments when some of us have to shut our eyes, it is the type of film that ultimately opens your eyes about the issue and the industry.

Today —— Rent and watch *Absolutely Safe*.

—•— 264 —•—

Find Three Things to Enjoy Today

Over the years, I have read Mary Pipher's books with great interest. *Reviving Ophelia* made me nod and tear up. *Writing to Change the World* had me taking copious notes. I held my hand to my mouth, recognizing myself in so many places, as I moved through *Seeking Peace*. As Pipher undergoes her own personal transformation after a meltdown, she seeks the best tools to help her find peace. One of those tools came from her Aunt Margaret, who watched as her husband of sixty years slipped away. Pipher writes, "Still, she managed to have fun and stay interested in the world. She told me her secret was to find three things to enjoy every day."

Today —— In your *Beautiful You* journal, reflect on three things that you took the time to enjoy today. Don't have three things? Reflect on the one or two things that you enjoyed. Now turn your attention to tomorrow. You can't possibly anticipate every enjoyable thing that will come your way because many wonderful moments are spontaneous, but go ahead and think about what you can enjoy tomorrow. You can help yourself anticipate a day that is tinged with joy.

— ◆ 265 ◆ —

Listen to Trisha

In the September 2009 issue of *Good Housekeeping,* Trisha Yearwood shares what she has learned about happiness. When asked what she would tell her younger self, here is how she answered:

> I spent a lot of time, especially in my 20s, stressing about my weight... I would love to go back and say to my young self, 'You waste so much time worrying about things that don't matter. Nobody ever said you're not going to get a record deal or a Grammy if you don't lose 20 pounds.' I got to do everything that I've ever wanted to do and beyond. So it wasn't about that for anybody else except for me.

Today ⟞ Consider Trisha's words and what they mean to your reality.

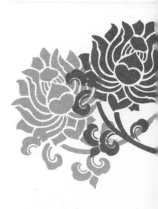

— 266 —

Love an Animal

We rescued Lola when she was four months old. Treated for mange, for worms, for parvovirus, our girl—possibly Australian shepherd mixed with all sorts of other breeds—was one sick puppy when we brought her home. When we walked into the house and put her down on our bedroom floor, we were overcome with a rank smell we hadn't noticed before.

"What is that?" we asked as we covered our noses. Turns out, it was our girl.

We bathed her four and five times a day for those first few days, but nothing changed. She still reeked. Then we noticed her lunge for a dead animal as she walked us, and we came to understand that the smell wasn't on her. It was in her.

Over the next few weeks, our mutual affection grew and her hunger for roadkill diminished. We'd rub her belly, stroke her nose, tug on her ears, and she'd press into us, begging for more. It didn't matter what kind of day we had had or what we looked like, Lola couldn't get enough of us. And that's the joy, isn't it, of loving an animal? They love you, no matter what, and they make you feel dramatically better.

Today — Enjoy an animal in your life. No pets at home? Borrow a friend's pet for a walk or a game of fetch. Or consider asking your local shelter about volunteer opportunities.

Speak Your Mind

One day, a few minutes before class, a student casually told me that a local bar had recently added a drink called a "Roofie Bomb" to its menu. A roofie, also known as the "date-rape drug," is a prescription form of Flunitrazepam, a hypnotic meant to treat severe cases of insomnia in the short term. Sadly, it has become the drug of choice for those who wish to sexually assault an unsuspecting person—they administer it by surreptitiously slipping it into a victim's drink, often at a bar. Just the week before in class, we had learned that the majority of sexual assaults happened while one or both parties were under the influence of alcohol. Couple that statistic with this menu addition, and my student's announcement just hung in the air like the affront that it was.

Later, I couldn't get the menu drink off my mind so I shot my student an email:

Hey Erin! I have thought about that roofie drink practically every day since you brought it up in class. I am not sure if you were planning on doing extra credit for class or not, but, if you are, I'd like to offer you extra credit for writing and sending that bar's headquarters a letter. I just think it is so important that we aren't silent when there is an issue that concerns us, and I always want to encourage my students and friends to speak up. If you are up for writing that letter, I am up for rewarding you for using your voice.

Erin quickly emailed me back:

It has been on my mind since I saw it, too! I have actually refused to go to that establishment (and it's one I frequent on a weekly basis for drinks with my girlfriends) until the drink is removed from the menu. That's one less patron than before, at least. I would absolutely love to write a letter for extra credit. I will provide you with a copy as soon as I get it typed up.

Silence is extremely damaging to our society. People don't speak out about things we know are wrong because we don't want to be "bitches" or go against a crowd, but in the end you have to decide if you want to be a follower or a leader. I want to be a leader and if being a "bitch" and speaking out is how I have to create change, I'm willing to do that for the greater good of our society and future.

I don't want my children to face what I face today, and change starts within institutions and with language. A drink called "Roofie Bomb" might sound innocent, but what is it saying about our views on rape and date rape? It's making it a joke and taking away from the seriousness of the crime. I'm glad to hear at least someone was bothered by it other than me. That means just by me making an off-handed statement, I changed or influenced one person; if everyone did that imagine how many people could be reached!

Today ⟶ Consider how much words matter. They influence us, change our minds, encourage us. Write a letter to a television show, magazine, movie, writer, or company that negatively portrays women or sends out a negative message about women. Let them know what you think. Remember Erin's words: *If everyone did that, imagine how many people could be reached.* And if you're wondering about how Erin's letter was received, the drink was immediately dropped from the menu.

— 268 —

Give Flowers

When I was a college administrator, one of the student groups I advised was looking for a new fundraiser. They wanted to provide a unique service or event that people would find irresistible. I had attended this same college as an undergraduate, and I remember being struck by the hundreds of tulips that popped up all over campus for most of the spring. Those flowers delighted me on my very first visit and continued to do so for years afterward, as an undergraduate and as an administrator.

As I was walking home one day, thinking about what we could do for an unusual fundraiser, the tulips popped into my mind. That spring, we launched Tulip Days—two weeks of daily flower deliveries. Recipients across campus received a bundle of ten tulips at their dorm room or office, with a note from the person who had sent them. What I realized during Tulip Days was that people enjoyed sending flowers just as much as they enjoyed receiving them. For both giver and receiver, it provided an incredible surge of joy and goodwill.

Today —— Stop by your local florist, grocery store, farmer's market, or field and gather some flowers to give to someone you love or appreciate.

— 269 —

Eat Slow

When we were kids, we had the following rule at our house: Eat what you want, but when you are done and want to be excused, you will go start the dishes.

I was the youngest and didn't really catch on to the fact that I could control whether or not I did the dishes. My sister, older and wiser, did. So she became a slow, deliberate eater who lingered over a meal, took breaks, enjoyed it, and could later recall what she'd eaten. In general, I am not that person.

Even now, Sonia still lingers over a meal and I still like to get the job done. At restaurants, she'll cut everything into bites and then slowly chew on a small forkful of food.

"We're at a restaurant," I'll insist, "you don't have to do the dishes here!" Still, she enjoys and experiences her meal rather than treat it like eating is just one more task in her day. Later, when I want ice cream, she is still sufficiently satisfied from the avocado she ate. Truth be told, she's likely on to something more than just how to skip out on the dishes.

Today —— Enjoy your meal. Put your fork and knife down between bites. Taste everything. *Linger*. Don't shovel. Let the meal be as sensational as it was meant to be.

— 270 —

Ask Yourself Three Questions

T aking pleasure in daily life greatly enhances one's sense of well-being. By candidly considering what is happening in life that is touching, and reflecting on whether or not we need to embrace more joyful possibilities, we begin to create beautiful lives of our imagining.

Today —— In your *Beautiful You* journal, answer these three questions with one-sentence answers. What surprised me today? What moved me today? What inspired me today?

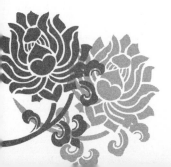

— 271 —

Wear Something Absurd

I was the type of girl who wasn't confident enough to wear a costume for the "Tacky Party" or whatever the theme party was in college. A few years later, as a teacher doing something that I loved and that I was good at, sporting a costume for Halloween was not at all a stretch. With a boom box in hand, my hat tipped sideways, and wearing oversized athletic wear, I wasn't afraid to delight my students with my impersonation of the gangsta' rappers they loved at the time.

Dressing up for Halloween made me realize that taking yourself too seriously can actually keep you from accessing confidence. It's when you are willing to laugh at yourself that you realize how debilitating self-seriousness can be. Taking yourself lightly can enhance your ability to embrace yourself and maintain a healthy perspective about life.

Today —— Wear something a little bit absurd. Maybe it's a funny bauble given to you by a friend, maybe it's a slightly loud shade of nail color, maybe it's a pair of funny shoes that will get noticed. Just wear it, check your ego at the door, and watch your brilliance shine as you get a kick out of yourself all day. Others will get a kick out of you too.

— 272 —

Listen to Henry

H enry Miller, an American author, wrote, "Develop interest in life as you see it; in people, things, literature, music—the world is so rich, simply throbbing with rich treasures, beautiful souls and interesting people. Forget yourself."

I fell in love with this quote when I was young. It appeared in my journals, on my vision boards, and danced around in my head. It has buoyed me with its truth and served as a reminder about the way forward.

Today ⟶ Appreciate the wisdom of Henry Miller's words.

Get Connected

With my tendency toward introversion, I can easily allow myself to go down the bunny hole of doing work, caring for my family, and forgetting to keep myself connected in my friendships. Yet staying connected brings me such joy, gives me access to support, allows me to be useful by offering support, expands my life, and provides a greater overall sense of satisfaction with my life. Oh, the irony!

Today —— Seek out a supportive friend for lunch, dinner, a walk, a phone conversation, coffee, dessert, a play date, or whatever fits into your schedule.

— 274 —

Try a Recipe with a Child in Your Life

Oh, food. Such an innocent little word, such a necessary part of our life, and such a loaded concept. Every semester in my body image class, I am struck by the damaging things heard around kitchens across America as families prepare, eat, or compensate for meals. Who are the people most internalizing those diet diatribes or ultimatums for love? Young people, who form solid ideas about health, nutrition, food, and beauty based on their parents' commentary in the central room of American homes.

Today —— Take back the power of the kitchen. Invite a child or young person in your life to create a meal—one that will bring nutritious benefit to all who share it—with you in your kitchen. Use an ingredient he or she has never tried, try a piece of equipment you rarely use, and enjoy the process of nurturing loved ones.

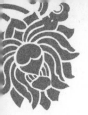

— 275 —

Schedule a Full Physical

P art of being body-confident is being in the know about your body. Unfortunately, too many of us put off important health screenings like cholesterol or blood-sugar tests. Women, especially, figure that if they visit their gynecologist regularly for their annual exam, they've covered all their bases. But unless your gynecologist does a full workup, you are missing valuable information about your health.

Today ⟶ Call your primary care physician and schedule a full physical. If you don't have a primary care physician, ask around for recommendations and do some research online. After you've scheduled your appointment, make a list of your concerns and questions so you can make the best use of your time with the doctor. Finally, remember that this commitment to yourself is part of actively celebrating your brilliance.

— 276 —

Know Your Family Health History

Being in the know about your body means you also know about historical health factors that might influence your well-being. Your quest to be body-and-soul confident does not end with your physical appointment. You also need to learn more about your own family's health history.

Today —— Now that you have that full physical scheduled, it's time to do your homework. If your biological parents are still alive, give them each a call and learn the details about the health challenges they face, as well as the health challenges that their parents and siblings faced. If your parents have passed away, contact your aunts, uncles, cousins, or grandparents to fill in the gaps.

If you were adopted, don't fret; there is still information that you can gather for your own health benefit. Talk to your parents to make sure that you accurately remember the details they have told you about your adoption story. You might hear new details about your biological parents that can be helpful. Also ask your family about illnesses or tendencies that you had when you were young. That information can be useful to your physician.

Know That the Journey Is the Goal

Recently, my friend Anna decided that she was going to train for and complete an Ironman race (2-mile swim, 112-mile bike ride, and 26.2-mile run). Anna had done some sprint triathlons before, as well as a couple marathons, so it wasn't outside the realm of possibility. But most Ironman participants will tell you that they spend a year or more preparing for the race. The catch: Anna decided to do it with just twenty weeks to spare. She did the research, learned what to do, and then did it.

Completing an Ironman is fairly bad-ass, but what I love about Anna's approach is that she didn't focus on the finish line. She savored the training journey. She loved how she felt every single day as she ate and practiced like an Ironman. I have never seen anyone have more fun training for something, and her spirit was always transparent. "Every day that I train is an accomplishment," she said to me.

Anna's approach is exactly right. Our world can be so result-oriented that we often forget that the process is what is important. It is the journey that is our reward. If we can enjoy the steps we take toward our goals, we will understand that the point isn't the finale but the lush crescendo in our lives as we journey toward it.

Today —— Consider any and all of the journeys you are currently taking. Can you relish each step and release your tight grip on what the outcome might be? Can your pleasure be the process?

Do Yoga

Yoga has many benefits outside of increased flexibility. Various studies have shown that yoga is a natural pain reliever; it boosts energy and improves mood. It reduces the level of cortisol, the body's stress hormone, which leads to a calmer mind; and it seems to induce mindful eating in its practitioners.

But did you know that yoga also seems to reduce body image anxiety in its practitioners? A study by Jennifer Daubenmier, published in a 2005 issue of *Psychology of Women Quarterly,* reveals that yoga's ability to help its practitioners develop body responsiveness—the ability to find just the right balance between a challenge and pain—actually decreases their likelihood of disordered eating and self-objectification. Yogis, in fact, felt better about their bodies than non-practitioners, and the longer a woman had been practicing yoga, the higher her self-esteem.

Today —— Do yoga. Take a class offered at a local studio or gym, do your own practice, pop in a yoga video, or find one on YouTube: just get your asanas on.

Complete This Sentence

Today you are just going to look at the positive, beautiful, miraculous things about your body.

Today ⟶ Open up your *Beautiful You* journal and complete this sentence with only positive thoughts.

My body is . . .

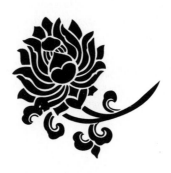

— 280 —

Ask for a Sign

I have had so many signs in my life. A phone call saying there was a baby boy who needed a family that came just an hour after I spoke with some friends about adoption. A supervisor's inadequate answers to questions about values that came just as I was deciding what my next professional step would be. An old house on my running route that I'd always loved going up for sale just after I said I really wanted to live in an old house.

When we look back at our lives, we see so many signs. Yet in the present, we often fail to ask for them, to let the universe or the God of our understanding know we are willing to be led. By offering up that we are paying attention, that we have a specific question in mind, that we are searching, we prepare ourselves for the answer that might be looking for us.

"It goes to the whole notion of not needing all the answers but trusting that the answers will find me when I need them," says spirituality writer Polly Campbell. "By asking for a sign, I am doing everything I can to get all the information. Sometimes I am not just asking, I am begging. I really think that developing the awareness enough to ask for something is prayer: give me the information I need or the people I need to show me what I should do. By asking for a sign, it puts you in that place of awareness and mindfulness and thinking about what you need and where you are. When you have the right question, it allows you to move forward into a place of possibility. With that said, signs might come in, but you may not like what's coming in. If you put it out there, you have to be open to all the possibilities. The whole experience is to grow, experience, love, and learn."

Today —— Whether through deliberate prayer or a question put out to the universe, ask for a sign.

— 281 —

Remember Those Beautiful Moments

A few years ago, I gave the keynote address at the Alpha Delta Kappa Southeastern Region Conference. Alpha Delta Kappa is an organization for women educators. The talk was on how to consciously develop sisterhood and understanding, and this dynamic, fun group of women was just the perfect audience for the conversation. After my talk, I signed books for over a hundred women and enjoyed brief conversations with each one of them. One woman shared that a friend of hers who'd recently had a baby was lamenting that she wasn't already back to her pre-pregnancy size. That little story broke my heart until the woman told me that she looked at her friend, incredulously, and said, "You have never been more beautiful than when you are talking to your daughter." What a beautiful thing to notice, and what a powerful compliment to share with a friend. That conversation took place a few years before I had my own child, but I now know that the woman in me that I love best is the woman who scoops up her baby boy each morning and whispers sweet things to him while he gingerly wakes up. I love that woman in me so much that even in her pajamas, with her unadorned face and crazy, wild, morning hair, she's beautiful to me.

Today —— If you are a parent, remember those tender, sweet moments you have had with your child. Let the tougher moments fall by the wayside so that all that is left are those sweet spots. If you are not a parent, consider a tender moment you have had with a child in your life. Bask in your beauty.

Chat Up Someone New

My introversion can sometimes be paralyzing, but I've learned over time that I gain something when I forge a connection with someone else. Maybe I form a lasting friendship. Maybe I learn something new. Maybe I make the right contact for a work or personal project. Maybe I just laugh in that moment or get a surge of joy that I didn't have before. By opening myself up to other people, especially people that I didn't necessarily know before, I enhance my own life, and enhancing my life leads to greater personal satisfaction.

Today — Meet someone new. It can be as simple as having a quick exchange in the elevator or talking for a moment to the delivery person who drops by with a package. By exhibiting the confidence you need to meet someone new, you are forging greater certainty in yourself.

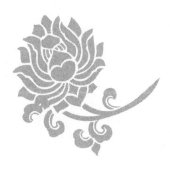

— 283 —

Read *The Vagina Monologues*

When I first read *The Vagina Monologues,* my soul sung in recognition. Eve Ensler was doing the work that I had dreamed of—listening to people's stories and compiling them in a way that allowed them to be heard, *really* heard, by others. Next, I saw *The Vagina Monologues* performed at the college where I worked, and I was further captivated by the power of the written word when spoken aloud. A year later, the student organizer of the campus production came to my office and asked me to be a part of the upcoming show.

"Absolutely," I said.

He breathed a dramatic sigh of relief. "Oh, thank God," he said. "There are a couple new monologues this year and when I read this one, I knew that you were the one person who could pull it off."

He handed me a monologue titled "My Short Skirt."

"My short skirt is not an invitation, a provocation, an indication that I want it, that I need it, or that I hook. My short skirt is not begging for it. It does not want you to rip it off me or pull it down...My short skirt, believe it or not, has nothing to do with you."

Fueled by its defiance, poise, clarity, and strength, I already felt the anticipation of getting on the stage and asserting myself for all of the women of the world. It was, indeed, my voice that Ensler captured in "My Short Skirt."

Today ⟶ Stop by your local library or bookstore and pick up a copy of *The Vagina Monologues,* then give yourself time to pour into them. As you read, consider which monologue was meant for you. When you're done, recite it with a firm conviction, owning each word as you give it voice.

— 284 —

Nap

When I was in college, I would sometimes allow myself to take what I called "a juicy nap"—a twenty-minute power nap. I always awoke from those juicy naps refreshed and with just the right amount of energy to push through the rest of my day. There were times when I would forego the nap, feeling it was an extravagance and I just needed to get on with my busy day. But I found that on days I didn't nap, I was never as eager, efficient, or joyful about the work still left before me. I almost didn't have the time *not* to nap.

Those naps were a caring gift to myself; making the effort to take them was a statement that I was making self-care a priority. And making yourself a priority is a significant part of the journey in celebrating one's brilliance.

Today —— Take a twenty-minute "juicy nap." You'll have excuses about why you can't, you'll worry about where to do it. Do it for yourself anyway. Worried you won't wake up, even with an alarm? Ask a friend to call you at a certain time. When you wake up, savor that refreshed feeling and notice how much better you function the rest of the day.

Be Quiet

We have become so accustomed to noise, to being constantly connected and plugged in, that we rarely relish the quiet anymore. Yet quietness, solitude, is really a gift, allowing us moments to cultivate self-awareness. It is in our quiet moments that we tune in and pay attention to ourselves and our needs. It is important to our well-being that we offer ourselves those quiet moments.

Today — Choose to be quiet for at least ten minutes. You can spend those minutes however you like: rocking on a chair on the porch, enjoying a cup of tea, etc. The key is to turn away from the world's chatter for a moment. By enjoying the solitude, you'll immediately feel peace and calm and a greater sense of well-being.

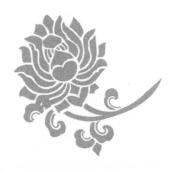

— 286 —

Write Your Six-Word Memoir

Legend has it that Ernest Hemingway was once challenged to write a story in only six words. The result: "For sale: baby shoes, never worn."

In 2006, Smith magazine issued a call for six-word memoirs and subsequently published a compilation of them in *Not Quite What I Was Planning*. The beauty of the six-word memoir is its powerful simplicity. In just six words, you can deliver humor, hope, poignancy, passion, and so much more. And the value of seeing your life distilled in such a simple form is that it brings clarity and perspective.

Today — In your *Beautiful You* journal, write your six-word memoir. Want to share it or need inspiration? Visit www.smithmag.net.

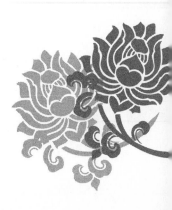

— 287 —

Add Color to Your Life

Vivid color has such a therapeutic effect. A flash of fuchsia or orange or aqua can boost our mood, bringing us joy with its pop.

Today ——— Incorporate color into your day. Wear a cranberry sweater, a lime scarf, red lipstick (well, maybe not all together). Bring color into your day and enjoy the boost it provides.

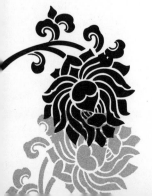

— 288 —

Stretch

I t is often when I fall into bed at night that I begin to feel the toll of the day: My back aches, my calves are tight, my shoulders are up by my ears. But I am lying in bed already, and I don't want to get out of bed to stretch. So instead I just lie there in pain, willing myself to sleep.

I was easily losing fifteen minutes of sleep to the tight, unhappy muscles in my body. When I realized this one day, I decided to use those fifteen minutes differently. Rather than ignore my body's needs all day and then have it demand my attention at night, I would spend some time stretching throughout the day. After just a few days of stretching, my body felt completely different by the end of the day—and I was able to sleep better.

Today —— Stretch for three minutes at a time, five times a day. If you need ideas about stretching, Google "daily stretches" and you'll find plenty of options. Pay particular attention to the parts of your body that get especially cranky by the end of the day. If you put in the time to acknowledge your body, you'll increase your range of motion and feel less (or no!) pain. When your body feels better, you feel better about your body.

Think of a Loved One

Ever notice that when you think about a loved one, you feel a greater sense of well-being? Reminding yourself that you are loved and that you love others brings forth feelings of joy, compassion, and contentedness.

Today —— When you find yourself obsessing over something negative, switch your thinking. Consciously think of a loved one and enjoy the feelings and emotions that arise.

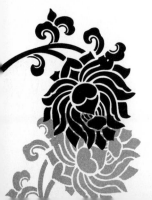

— 290 —

Reconnect with an Old Friend

The subject line on the email read: My Favorite Picture.

The email itself read:

I was cleaning out the drawers of a dresser I'm getting rid of and I came across my favorite picture of you: little girl in a soccer uniform, full-on scowl, and a look in your eyes like you want to bite the cameraman's ear off. The contrarian in me always liked seeing the sweetest girl I've ever met looking like a total bad-ass.

The email landed in my in-box just months after I became a new mom. I had long forgotten that picture, which shows that I hated being photographed even in second grade. When the email arrived, I was dulled from a chronic lack of sleep, and I had forgotten that I was ever the sweetest girl anyone had ever met. Not that I wasn't nice during that time as a new mother; I was just so tired that I couldn't even remember who I was.

This email was from one of my closest high school friends, a guy I have many fond memories of and who knew me so well by the time we graduated. It only reached me because we had reconnected almost two years before. I was getting ready to travel to Chicago to promote *Hijas Americanas,* and I had decided to look him up. In Chicago, it was easy to be with him again after so many years. While I knew how much I had loved him, it was nice to be reminded—by someone who knew me at my core—about what was loveable about me.

We can reconnect with old friends through social media like MySpace, Facebook, and Twitter. Old friends put us back in touch with our true selves. They can remind us of who we are at our core, when jobs, marriage, children, and the like are peeled away from us. And sometimes we need that reminder, that jolt of "Oh, yeah, I'm sweet" when we are feeling anything but.

Today —— Look up an old friend and get in touch. Remember who you were when you knew that person, how that essence is still in you, and how far you have come.

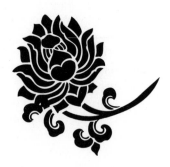

Drink Tea

Though I don't do it often enough, I have found that drinking hot tea makes me feel both indulgent and virtuous—like I am doing something terribly sophisticated while taking care of my body.

Today ——◂ Every time you want a cup of coffee or a can of soda today, have a cup of hot tea instead. For an added bonus, opt for green tea. It contains L-theanine, which is believed to have a calming effect on the mind.

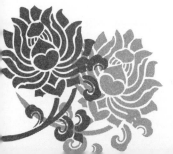

— 292 —

Realize That We All Feel Like "the Other"

The uniqueness of the human experience is that we each have a mind, and thus, an inner dialogue that accompanies us as we go through life. What our mind notices is part of what makes us unique; it illuminates how we are different from others. The reality, though, is that sometimes we perceive we are more different, more alone, more "the other" than anyone else.

Today —— Consider the fact that we are all unique; hence, we all feel like "the other" at moments in our lives. The beauty of the human experience is that we are each uniquely made.

DAY

293

Generate Good Karma

Sometimes we can get a simple boost of joy and a sense of well-being from discretely doing something that is good for someone else.

Today — Generate some good karma. The next time you pull in to the shopping center and see a primo parking spot, drive by it and let someone else experience the joy of snagging a killer spot when she arrives at the grocery store. Or let someone go in front of you in line. The flush of goodness you will feel is grounding, and the goodwill you will generate for yourself is satisfying.

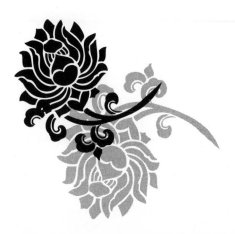

327

DAY

— 294 —

Take Your Pulse

Getting a feel for how you are doing and where things stand in your life at the moment is a valuable tool in moving forward.

Today — In your *Beautiful You* journal, answer these questions: What are you feeling right now? What does it mean? Why are you feeling it? How do you feel about it?

Mind Your Posture

When we see a person with poor posture, we wonder if the slump in her spine is because of apathy or lack of confidence. Our body language says so much about us, and our most prominent body language is arguably our posture. Standing tall projects confidence and self-possession. When we change the message people receive from us, we change the message they give us back.

Today —— Mind your posture by holding your body erect and your head high. Push those shoulders down and back and revel in the confidence you feel as you project a stronger front.

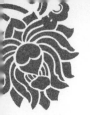

— 296 —

Walk Whenever Possible

I live in a walkable town. It is one of the features of my small town that I love the most. So you would think I would take more advantage of it, but I don't. I constantly work until the last possible minute, which forces me to drive to the coffeehouse where I have a meeting. I do the same thing when it comes to getting the last dinner ingredient I need or getting to the bank to deposit a check before it closes. I push myself to the brink in everything I do, and then I miss out on the perk I love most in my hometown.

Old habits are hard to break, but when I do allow myself to finish up my work in time to walk where I need to go, I am infinitely more satisfied and have a greater sense of well-being. Walking allows me to enjoy the day, visit with neighbors, think about something that has been in the back of my mind, and strategize for later.

Today — Walk whenever possible and enjoy its many benefits.

— 297 —

Follow a Theme

Years ago, I traveled to Scotland and exhausted my camera with snapshot after snapshot. Back home, with the photos developed, I struggled over which photos to place in a photo album and which to place in a frame. I wanted a framed photo of a sheep, but all of them were so beautiful and had something unique that I especially liked. This one had a black spot in the midst of its white coat, that one had a funny look on its face. The same held true for my photos of headstones in the centuries-old cemetery, of window boxes in every small town we visited, and the brightly colored doors in Edinburgh or Inverness. When I looked at those photos, I lost myself in the details and loveliness of each one.

The metaphor here isn't much of a stretch. Each of us assigns value to our appearance and our skills; we see them as better than or less than those of other people, not simply different. And yet, my photographs, which I'd piled up by themes, showed me that there is no "better than." Things are simply different—not better than, not less than, just wholly unique. None of us are meant to be exactly alike.

Today ⸺ Follow a theme with your camera. Snap photos of flowers, birds, mushrooms, children, window boxes, doorknobs, or whatever you like. Later, look over the images you've collected and notice the lovely details that make each one unique.

— 298 —

Sing Out Loud

There is something about belting out a tune that just makes me happy. Music can be so cathartic—the lyrics speak to us, the rhythm moves us; when we sing, we feel heard and understood. When a song resonates with us, we feel less like "the other" and less alone.

Today —— Think of a song that has particular meaning to you and sing it at any opportunity—in the shower, while getting ready for your day, in the car, while cooking dinner. Hear those words roll around in your head, feel the music within and savor that sensation, and understand that your experience is not foreign; you are not alone.

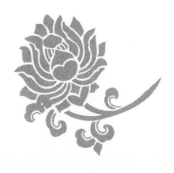

— 299 —

Take a Child to a Playground

One of the great joys of childhood is arriving at a playground or park and seeing infinite possibilities for fun. At parks and playgrounds, kids learn how to enjoy the way their bodies move. They are treated to surprises and joys that happen nowhere else. Those early messages inform our children for a lifetime. By providing them more opportunities to play and move, we give them more power over their bodies and greater understanding that there is delight in movement.

Today ⸺ Take a child to a playground. Don't just sit on a park bench while she frolics; follow along and engage in her play. You will laugh and have new experiences, and both of you will leave fully satisfied.

— 300 —

Spend Money on Someone Else

R etail therapy. Many of us have tried using it to make us feel better, yet very few of us have had successful results. The thrill we get from that new sweater is fleeting, likely because shopping doesn't automatically tap into our best selves.

That said, a group of researchers at the University of British Columbia did find a way to feel better after spending money: spend it on someone else. In a 2008 study published in the journal *Science,* the researchers found that spending money on other people has a more positive impact on happiness than spending money on yourself. The even better news? All it took was $5 to feel a boost from your generosity.

Today —— Take a friend out to lunch or coffee or pick up a simple surprise for someone while you are out and about. Then enjoy the surge of goodness you feel as a result of your generosity.

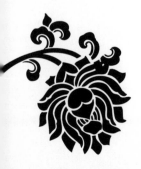

— 301 —

Schedule Some Skin Time

When we are self-conscious about our bodies, we become more reluctant to do the necessary self-exams that could save our lives. Sometimes we are hesitant to be naked—even with just ourselves as witness. But taking care of your body boosts your sense of self. And taking care of your body's largest organ—your skin—can also have a tremendous impact on your long-term health.

Today —— Schedule an annual skin exam with a dermatologist. Ask your primary care physician or your friends for a referral, or find one using your insurance company's provider book. Next, open your calendar and schedule monthly appointments with yourself to complete skin self-exams. Schedule them for the rest of the year, and get started today by doing this month's check. Visit www.cancer.gov/cancertopics/wyntk/skin/page13 for instructions on how to perform a skin self-exam.

— 302 —

Take a Break Before Speaking

I am ashamed to say that there have been times in my life where I have said an unhelpful or hurtful thing because I didn't consider my words before saying them. After those moments, I have felt the sting of what I said just as surely as the person who heard it did. When we consider our words, we help create more positive possibilities. There is a difference between telling someone "You drink entirely too much" and saying, "I am worried about you." And that difference is significant in both the short term and the long term.

Today —— Take a break before speaking. Consider your words and the context of your situation. Ask yourself if what you are adding to the conversation is helpful, true, and clear, and if the way you plan to present it is respectful. Then proceed.

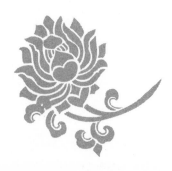

— 303 —

Get a Mentor

O ver the course of my life, I have been blessed with wonderful mentors. Some of them were personal mentors, others were professional mentors. All of them helped me act more deliberately, make better informed choices, and grow. What I learned by watching and talking to them is invaluable. I am a better person for having been guided by each one of them.

Today —— In your *Beautiful You* journal, consider two questions. First, what is the most pressing question in your life right now. (Some possibilities: What should I major in? Should I study abroad? What type of work do I want to do? Will I be happy in this field? How can I advance? What can I do to be a better mother?) Next, what person in your life do you most admire for the way she has handled that question for herself? Reach out to that person and seek some practical advice.

DAY

— 304 —

Use Your Frustration

Feeling like we've hit a wall can be maddening, but frustration is actually a valuable tool in the journey to self-actualization and confidence. Frustration is a signal that we are dissatisfied with a situation and something needs to change. Yes, you are in a tough position, but you also have an opportunity to change the situation for the better and to grow.

Today —— Consider a recent frustration. How can you use the experience as an opportunity to create change and grow? If you need some perspective, talk to someone with experience in that area. Then use the frustration to move you toward something that is healthier, more productive, and more authentic for you.

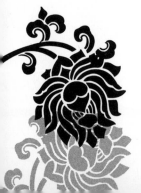

— 305 —

Take a Silent Hike with a Friend

Sometimes, being out in nature offers us the most powerful insights. Taking time out to enjoy the outdoors is grounding and gives us time to gain some clarity in that moment.

The stress-reducing effects of nature can be seen rather quickly, according to Dr. Jolina Ruckert, a researcher in developmental psychology at the University of Washington. "With nature, it's just as much about the quality as the quantity. It's not just about how much time you spend in nature, but what you do when you're there. Engaging all the senses is important: touching the earth, smelling the scents, listening to the sounds. This is more a personal commitment—not being afraid to get dirty; pushing personal, physical, and psychological boundaries; being confronted with the uncomfortable. Nature can offer these powerful experiences. Jump into a cold lake. Hike a small mountain. Stand at the edge of the cliff. Encounter a wild animal. I'm not suggesting death-defying feats in nature, but a recognition that being in nature can offer one to move outside their comfort zones, push boundaries, feel humility, see its beauty, and grow in the experience."

Today —⌐ Make a date to go on a hike with a friend and then tackle a local trail in silence. The silence will offer you the opportunity for thoughtful reflection. Enjoy the scenery, push yourself and engage your senses, and on the way home, talk through the experience and any epiphanies you may have had. Need help finding a local hike? Visit www.localhikes.com.

— 306 —

Take a Personal Health Day

We are often as productive as possible every single day, not leaving much room for relaxation or self-care. But by giving ourselves a day of nurturing—whether it's a weekend day or weekday—we get back in touch with ourselves and recharge.

Today — Schedule a personal health day. What would your ideal day look like? Fresh berries for breakfast on the porch? Reading in bed? A long bath or nap? Whatever a personal health day looks like to you, treat yourself to experiencing it for at least one day.

— 307 —

Cross a Finish Line

Afew years ago my dad was diagnosed with lymphoma. While we were processing that news, one of my best friends called to say her son had Hodgkin's disease.

I flew to Texas to be with my friend and her family. I drove to Columbia and watched doctors aspirate marrow from my father's hip with a needle the size of my forearm, the first step on his way to treatment. My world shrank in the face of cancer, and the road between my house and my parents' house narrowed. I sent cards to my dad that arrived every day during his treatment. I e-mailed doctors, read medical journals, learned about environmental hazards near my parents' house, researched cancer clusters. My world was consumed with the chronicling of a sickness.

Eventually, the passivity that's part of being a family member during the treatment process (the sit and wait, the watch and wonder) was more than I could bear. The small actions that I had assigned myself—the reading, calling, questioning—were not enough. I had to move, and my movement had to change the count of those who were succumbing to cancer.

Although I was a cycling novice, I signed up for a 100-mile bike ride and fundraiser in honor of my dad and my friend's son. I would use this "century ride" to raise money for Team in Training, a fundraising program for The Leukemia and Lymphoma Society (LLS).

When the first race finished, I signed up for another. For me, each pedal stroke propelled me toward beating cancer. Each mile had a price, and that price was life. I may not have been a natural athlete, but I was spinning at my breakneck best to change the count. Crossing those finish lines connected me to something larger than myself and it also connected me to the power of my own body.

As a friend once said to me, once you cross a finish line, you enter a whole new frontier, a place you have never been. Still today, the feelings I experienced as I crossed various finish lines stay with me and inform my sensibilities. Once you cross a finish line, once you have challenged yourself to go further or faster than you thought possible, you realize everything changes. You have challenged yourself to train for something and accomplish it. You learn just what you have in you, and you never go back to the time when you doubted what was possible.

Today —— Sign up to cross the finish line of your choice. By engaging in an athletic journey, whether or not it is attached to a fundraising mission, you are moving for your own survival and honoring your body and its abilities.

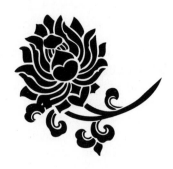

— 308 —

Love a Child Who Is Not Your Own

We all had adults who cared about us when we were young who were not our parents—a coach, a teacher, a youth minister. Kids need more people on their team than just their parents. There comes a point in every kid's life where she begins to think that her parents are just saying those nice things because they are supposed to, "since they're my parents and all." That's when a mentor makes even more of a difference. Every child, regardless of the size of her allowance or house, needs a cadre of people who care about her in her life. And part of becoming our best selves is actively sharing what we have to offer.

Today —— Think about how you might be able to help care for a child who does not live in your house. Do you have the time and energy right now to be a mentor? If so, look for mentoring organizations in your community, such as Big Brothers Big Sisters. Can you pull an extra ornament off an Angel Tree at the holidays? Can you make a contribution to an organization that champions kids? How about signing up to teach an afterschool class in your area of expertise? (Check out www.citizenschools.org if this option is interesting to you.) Will you agree to serve as a board member for a nonprofit that needs you? Decide how you can make a difference and then commit yourself. It will make as big a difference in your life, too.

— 309 —

Intervene on Someone Else's Behalf

Size, body, and beauty prejudice are actually related to all other types of discrimination. Recently, during a discussion about race, ethnicity, culture, class, and religion in the body image seminar I teach, a student shared an experience she'd had just days before.

"I was walking to class and a girl walked by me who was Muslim," Lauren relayed, explaining that the young woman was wearing a *hijab,* or head covering.

A male student, someone Lauren recognized as a member of the class she was walking to, passed the young woman. Just as he was reaching Lauren, he screamed at the woman, "I can still see you!"

Stunned and angry, Lauren turned to him, not worrying that she was about to spend an hour and a half sitting near him in class.

"Wow," she said confidently, in a matter-of-fact way. "You're an ass."

The young man was silent, but inside, I am certain he was reeling. When someone makes such a public attack, he is hoping to boost his image. He wants people to think that he is fearless and opinionated. Lauren's words brought him back down to earth, hopefully teaching him—and others—that discriminating against someone does not make you cool. It just makes you look pathetic.

Today —— Intervene on someone else's behalf. Work to identify and resist all forms of discrimination and stand up for those who have no power or voice in a particular situation. By raging against all forms of discrimination, more of us can be appreciated for exactly who we authentically are.

— 310 —

Order Dessert

few years ago, my husband and I went out to a very late dinner with friends. I had eaten something earlier in the evening to tide me over until dinner—a sandwich made with one piece of bread. (This is something I learned that my husband's grandfather used to do before evening weddings; he'd call it is his "foldover." Now, I call it my holdover.) When we arrived at the restaurant, I wasn't really hungry for a meal. I was, however, hungry for dessert. So while everyone else ordered roasted chicken, ribs, and steak, I ordered strawberry shortcake as my entree. It was fabulous, and I enjoyed every bite.

Food. We have worked it over so much in our brains that ordering something at a restaurant is now a hotbed of dos and don'ts. And while I think eating healthfully and mindfully is really important for keeping our bodies running their best, I also think that living in balance calls for the occasional indulgence.

Today —— Order dessert. Don't talk about it. Don't validate why you can have it. Just enjoy it.

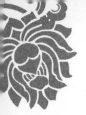

Stay Current

Part of getting over ourselves involves getting out of our minds and changing our focus; we must move from being me-centered to being other-centered. One great way to do that is to begin learning more about the world around you.

Today ⟞ Pick up a newspaper—not just an online edition but an actual printed newspaper—and read through it. Look at every story on every page and take in what is happening around your community, your country, and the world. Choose one news story that you'd like to continue to follow. Regularly—perhaps daily—seek out more information on the topic or issue in newspapers or on the Internet. By broadening your worldview, you move the focus away from your own worries and insecurities and begin to see the bigger picture.

— 312 —

Create a Study Guide to Your Body

We often know exactly what the people in our lives need. But we don't always know what *we* need, especially physically. You can learn more about your physical needs by creating an operating guide to your body.

Today — In your *Beautiful You* journal, draw yourself (from head to toe) in whatever way that you are most comfortable. Now, write a descriptive guide to operating your body. For example, you might draw an arrow pointing to your lower back and write "Happiest when stretched." Or draw an arrow to your legs and write, "Loves a good massage and long walks."

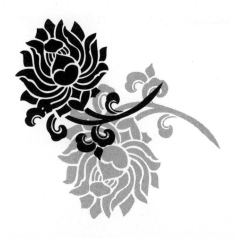

— 313 —

Meditate

While it might sound New Agey to some, meditation is laced with benefits. It has been shown to improve sleep, ease anxiety, and lower blood pressure and heart rate as it improves your sense of well-being and happiness. The best part? All it takes to reap these benefits is your commitment to making time for a calm moment—you aren't dependent on any external or environmental factors, nor do you need to force a tangible outcome. By just doing it, you give yourself a gift.

"I found it beneficial to be in a quiet dark space by myself. It took a longer time for me to find it beneficial on a spiritual level," reflects spirituality writer Polly Campbell. "You are giving yourself a time to sit and just be with your spirit. I do feel more centered, and I feel physically healthier—sometimes we just need to stop, sit down, and be quiet."

Today ⟿ Meditate for at least five minutes. Go to a quiet room, turn the lights down low, sit down, and close your eyes. Focus your awareness on your breath. Breathe in and out through your nose, slowing your breath and making it deeper. Next, guide yourself in releasing tension and letting go by concentrating on each body part and feeling that release, moving from head to feet. When you are done, linger for a moment as you consider how the exercise made you feel.

DAY

— **314** —

Create

It is so satisfying to create something that didn't exist before your hands put it together. We take disparate things, we bring them together, we mix them and coordinate them and manipulate them, and soon our unique fingerprint has been manifested in a collage, a painting, a poem, a song, a thank-you note, an aromatic slice of bread.

The value in creation goes beyond the end product—the birdhouse we built or the hat we crocheted. It is in the process—the active meditation as we build, the thought process that lets us take a sliver of a notion from the right side of the brain and make it into a concrete thing using the left side. It is in the engagement and concentration and revelation of what we can accomplish. And it is in the satisfaction we feel when we are finished.

Today —— Create something. Whether it is a loaf of bread or a scarf or a small watercolor, bring something into the world that was not previously here and bask in it.

— 315 —

Visit a Farm

Connecting to the earth and acknowledging the way it nurtures us is a powerful experience. Moreover, eating tasty farm-fresh food makes it easier for us to nurture our bodies. Local food changes hands less often and doesn't require processesing that diminishes its nutritional value. When we show our bodies care by putting only the best, freshest foods into it, we feel a greater sense of well-being.

Today ⟶ Visit a local farm where you can pick up (or pick!) fresh produce. Find a farm at www.pickyourown.org. If there isn't a farm nearby that welcomes visitors, consider participating in a community garden.

DAY

— 316 —

Simplify

It is hard to be our best selves when we are stuck in trappings that keep us contained in some way. I have found that when my space is cluttered, my mind is cluttered. When I am too distracted by the stimulation around me, I cannot be the person I want to be.

Today — First, consider whether the stuff in your life is getting in your way. Take out your *Beautiful You* journal, identify the clutter that exists in your life, and describe how it hinders you.

Next, get some of that stuff out of your way. Choose just one area of your home or office to declutter, with a mission of creating a streamlined space that can actually serve who you are right now. Grab a trash bag for things that need to be thrown away, a bag for recycling, a box for give-aways, and designate an area to put items you want to keep. Need some help? Call a discerning friend who can push you to really give up things you don't need. When you are done, make sure all the castaways get to where they need to go.

Now sit back and look around your room. Relish in the flow you feel now that the space surrounding you has been tamed.

— 317 —

Applaud an Effort

Just as it is important to express your opinion about campaigns or products that diminish women and our value, it is also important to express gratitude for efforts that celebrate our humanity in positive ways.

Today —— Write a letter to a television show, magazine, movie, writer, or company that positively portrays women and looks at beauty through more than one narrowly focused lens. Let them know what you think.

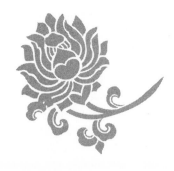

DAY

— 318 —

Eat a Meal with Your Hands

I n Ethiopia, meals are eaten by hand. *Injerra*, a flat bread that is similar to Indian *naan* or a tortilla, is the vehicle for bringing bits of stewed vegetables or meat dishes to a diner's lips. The tactile experience can make meals seem more sensational and satisfying.

Today —— Eat a meal with your hands, savoring the feel of each texture as you eat. If you enjoy various cuisines, you might try dining at an Ethiopian or Indian restaurant, where eating with the hands is common.

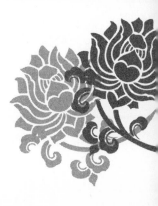

— 319 —

Walk a Labyrinth

Some people use the words *labyrinth* and *maze* interchangeably, but they are not quite the same thing. Mazes are often puzzles, with participants expected to make choices about the path and direction they take. Labyrinths typically have just one path, which leads to the center. It is one simple route, to the center and back, meant to be done as a walking meditation, and its rewards can be plentiful.

Catherine Anderson, a Charlotte, North Carolina–based artist, was so moved by the power of labyrinths that she built one in her backyard, just outside her studio. Her goal is to walk it every day.

"I use it as a meditative practice," Anderson says. "I can forget about where I have to go—I don't have to think about it—and that allows me to let go of a lot of stuff as I start to walk it. I don't have to think about where to go next. The labyrinth allows me to become almost meditative, but my body is still doing something.

"On the way in, I let go of the shopping list or 'do I have enough time to do this' thoughts," she continues. "Because it is outdoors, I can feel the wind or sun on my face or the grass under my feet. With this comes a tremendous amount of gratitude. For me, that gratitude makes me aware of the fact that I have my health, that I can walk around this labyrinth, that I can hear the birds, that I can see the leaves moving. It makes me very aware of the things that I am able to sense and feel through my physical body. I have never had a walk around the labyrinth where I come out thinking 'you are not tall enough' or 'your stomach is too big.' It almost seems like a connection to something larger than me, where I realize that what I look like is not really important; it is who I am that is important."

Today ⟿ Walk a labyrinth. Visit www.labyrinthlocator.com to find one near you. As you begin the walk, let go of all expectation and just focus on making the journey. "Just walk it quietly and mindfully and see what happens," says Anderson. "When you do anything mindfully, you let go of your judgments about yourself. You take the focus away from yourself."

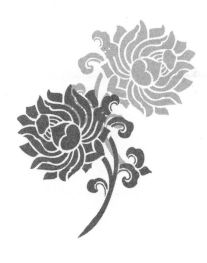

Consider These Words

When I interviewed artist Catherine Anderson about her labyrinth, we had a heartfelt conversation about body image issues: when they start, what causes them, and how to step away.

"It's about becoming so consumed by life and your talents and gifts and everything else that the importance of your body and how you imagine it should look falls away," I said.

"Yes," Catherine answered. "When all you are focusing on is yourself, it is easy to become enmeshed in that. When you have a passion, something that you just have to do, all of a sudden that self stuff falls away."

The day after our interview, I sat down to find this delightful quote from Catherine. The quote had landed in her inbox earlier that morning. It reminded her of me and this book, so she sent it my way.

Today —— Consider these words from Khalil Gibran: *Beauty is not in the face; beauty is a light in the heart.*

— 321 —

Reflect on Possibilities

We talked earlier about signs, about being open to being led in our lives. Today, we'll consider that idea further.

Today ⟶ In your *Beautiful You* journal, reflect on this question: What are the things, places, experiences, and people in your life that have helped you see new possibilities?

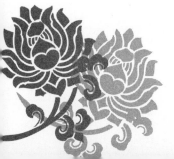

DAY

— 322 —

Affirm Your Image

Y ou already know that I don't love being photographed. I can argue that photographs are reductive, burning into permanence just one moment in time as seen through just one lens, making a multi-dimensional person two-dimensional. But I probably need to get over myself and realize that no one looks at pictures of me with as sharp an eye as I do. So, in the spirit of tackling my own demons (and knowing I am not the only woman who wishes never to have her picture taken again), I decided that the best way to end the reign of terror photos have over me would be to face a camera head-on. Kind of like someone who has a snake phobia might have to hold one to get to the other side of her fear.

On the day we met our baby boy for the first time, my husband had the camera ready. I wanted so much to say, "Only take pictures of the baby." But then I thought how sad it would be to not have photos of us all together on our first day as family. So I bit my tongue and let the camera roll. As it turned out, the photos from that day are some of my favorite photos ever—not because I look like a supermodel in them, but because I look exactly like what I was: an in-love new mother finding her way.

Today —— Snap (or have someone else snap) five pictures of you. They can be taken at different times of the day, while you are doing different things, or taken all at one time and in one place. Just get yourself to the other side of your fear and concentrate solely on letting a part of your interior essence show on the film. Are you joyful? Let it seep through onto the lens. Afraid? Sad? Hopeful? Whatever you are, share it with the lens in candid or posed photos and affirm the image that is yours alone.

— 323 —

Hear a Story

One of my favorite teaching assignments is asking my students to interview older family members about their life stories, or even about their body image. By hearing other people's stories, we gain an additional lens through which to look at our own lives. We also give our loved ones the joy of being listened to, which is an invaluable gift to give, one that's wonderful to realize we are capable of giving.

StoryCorps is a nonprofit oral-history project with a mission to honor and celebrate the lives of Americans from all backgrounds. Since it was established in 2003, tens of thousands of people have interviewed their friends and family members and shared their stories through StoryCorps. The project gives us the opportunity to experience the history, hopes, and humanity of those we love and those we have never met.

Today — Visit www.storycorps.org and lose yourself in the stories of others. By allowing ourselves to learn from others' experiences, by opening our hearts to what we hear, we also open our hearts to ourselves.

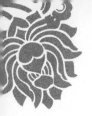

Watch *Bigger, Stronger, Faster*

omen think we're the only ones with body issues, but that's not the case at all. Boys and men are also desperately trying to fulfill an ideal that they perceive is universal and necessary. Why does this matter to us? Because we sometimes perpetuate it, because we raise and mentor boys, because some of us are partnered with men, because we are sisters and friends, and because we continue to cripple ourselves with these standards the more universal they become.

Today ——◦ Rent and watch *Bigger, Stronger, Faster*. This documentary is directed by Chris Bell who, along with his two brothers, has been a long-time powerlifter and bodybuilder. They started as boys who idolized Hulk Hogan, Sylvester Stallone, and Arnold Schwarzenegger, and they did everything they could in the weight room to be like their heroes. Except that their heroes were getting juiced with steroids. In the world of body-building, what you see is not always what you get (much like the world of advertising, where the bodies featured in advertisements are often air-brushed to perfection). The film shows Bell at a crossroads, interviewing athletes, physicians, parents, magazine editors, and students. Then he looks into the politics and psychology of steroids. Throughout the film, Bell explores questions about what we do to gain the competitive edge— and the cultural "norm" we then create with our behaviors.

DAY

— 325 —

Give a Girl a Journal

started journaling regularly when I was in middle school. When I talk about it now in the journaling workshops I lead, I often comment that journaling was the thing that kept me safe. It might sound like an exaggeration, but it's not. Journaling kept me safe because it kept me plugged into my voice. I always knew what I was thinking, and knowing what I thought kept me safe from what other people thought. It also made it harder for me to make choices that went against what my soul knew was right.

Today ⟶ Give a girl in your life a journal so she can capture her thoughts. Teach, encourage, and celebrate the unique voice and stories she has to share with the world. Owning her experience will keep her from giving that power to someone else.

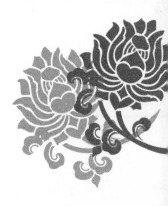

— 326 —

Work Your Brain

We spend so much time thinking about working the muscles all over our bodies that we sometimes forget to work our brains. Working our brains helps us feel more confident in our abilities and wards off diseases like dementia and Alzheimer's.

Today — Add ten minutes of mental exercise to your day. Flip to your local paper's puzzle page to tackle Sudoku, the crossword, and/or the word puzzles; visit an online site that offers your challenge of choice; or buy a book with mental exercises. By training your brain, you grow more confident in your problem-solving abilities, which means you grow more confident in yourself.

— 327 —

Be Harmonious

We are our most beautiful when we are perfectly in harmony with who we are.

Today —— In your *Beautiful You* journal, consider what makes you *you*. How can you be in better harmony with who you are?

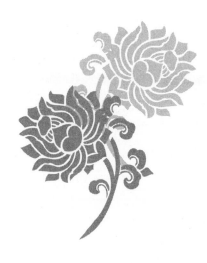

— 328 —

Don't Settle

Are you tempted to settle a little bit too much when it comes to finding a partner? If so, it's time to really think about what you want in a partner, and what the deal breakers are. When you go into a relationship just grateful that someone wants to be with you, you can lose sight of how important it is that this person is someone who brings out the best in you and who enriches your life. Relationships are hard work, even during the best of times, and being with a partner who doesn't enhance your life can quickly make it the worst of times.

Today —— Not in a relationship? In your *Beautiful You* journal, make a list of what you want in your partner and what your deal breakers are. Also, reflect on times when you have been happy in a relationship and analyze why. You don't have to follow your lists to the letter when choosing a partner, but they should help you recognize when you are settling in a relationship rather than expanding yourself through one.

If you are in a relationship, reflect on what compromises you are making in it (and there are always compromises in relationships). Are you okay with those compromises? If you feel like you are giving in too much, consider seeing a counselor to talk things over.

— 329 —

Have a Dinner Party

Every month, I look forward to two regular dinner parties. The first is dinner with my book club. There are six of us in this group, which came together organically, and we rotate hosting our dinner and discussion (which sometimes focuses on the book for about ten minutes before shifting to the rest of our lives and the world around us). The meals are always delicious, but the company is even better. When I pull out of the driveway or wash the last dish at my house, I do so with my well refilled.

The other dinner that makes my heart sing is a regular Scrabble dinner I host for two women who have been in my life since I was in college and who are wonderful mentors to me. I cook for them and then we sit around the table talking about movies, books, and what's going on in the neighborhood. Then we begin talking smack as the Scrabble board comes out and we put on our competitive faces. Those meals leave me equally content.

Sharing great meals are a way to strengthen our ties to each other. They help us to live more fully, to connect more deeply, to share some of our most crucial needs with others. They build community and foster our creativity. They boost our spirits.

Today ⊱—— Plan a dinner party in your home for one other person or several other people sometime in the upcoming week. Call and invite them, establishing a personal connection for the evening right then. Plan a menu that will bring you joy, and then begin working on it. Sharing a meal with loved ones will buoy your spirit and remind you that the experience of life is one that has very little to do with your appearance.

— 330 —

Take a Field Trip

The first time I went to a movie by myself, I was out of town and locked out of the place where I was staying. I could have gone shopping during that time, or sat in a coffeehouse and read a book, but I really wanted to see a movie, and I could rarely justify taking the time to do it. So I decided to forget the conventional wisdom that movie-going is a communal experience.

Rarely, it seems, do we go places we'd like to go if it means we have to do it alone. We don't go to movies alone, we hesitate trying a new restaurant we've been eyeing with a book as our sole companion, and we seldom visit a museum's new exhibit without someone with us. But we should, and for so many reasons—because we might not ever get the chance to go otherwise, because we experience things in a unique way when we experience them alone, because we deserve the nurturing and attention.

Today —— Treat yourself to an excursion. Whatever place might make your soul glad, go there alone and delight in it.

DAY

— 331 —

Consider What You've Gained

Y ou have been on this journey to awareness for almost a year. Hopefully, you have gained some tangible rewards for your effort.

Today —— In your *Beautiful You* journal, consider what you have gained in each of these areas: awareness, love, security, confidence, purpose, health, community, spirituality, joy.

Encourage a Girl in Your Life to Find Her Passion

One thing I saw clearly when I was writing *Hijas Americanas* was that the women who had found something they loved at a young age—gymnastics, skating, softball, soccer, writing, playing violin, singing, art, etc.—were the women who managed to escape adolescence without significant insecurities about who they were, how they looked, and what they had to offer. Developing proficiency in an activity boosts a girl's self-confidence and helps her find value in something other than how she looks. She understands that her body is a vehicle meant to allow her to enjoy life, not an object to be admired. Having a passion also gives her something to focus on when negative choices are presented to her later.

Today ⊶ Encourage a girl in your life to enjoy or find her passion. If she already knows what she loves, ask her about it. Put her sports games on your calendar and go cheer her on. Admire her artwork. Engage in whatever she loves so she can see what she has to offer. If she doesn't yet know what she loves, encourage her to explore her interests and help her think through what she might want to embrace. You will be reminding yourself of a valuable lesson while teaching her one as well.

DAY

— 333 —

Realize That It Is Impossible to Satisfy Everybody

Has there been a moment (or seventy) in your life where you have tried hard to make everybody around you happy? You've cooked the multi-course meal so that everybody's favorites are on the table; you've given up what you needed to get done on a Saturday so that everybody else's wants could be met; you've smiled away your preferences so someone else could be happy. You feel so good about going without, about meeting every-body's needs, and then *voila!* You find that still, despite your best efforts, no one is happy: The gravy's too runny, the movie wasn't funny enough, the day did not go as someone else wanted. And there you are, licking the colossal wounds that have been left—the ones delivered in blows because you failed to satisfy everybody else's needs and the ones delivered in whis-pers because, deep down, you knew the whole time you were selling your-self out to buy someone else's joy. And it didn't work.

Today —— Realize that it is impossible to satisfy everybody. So temper the people-pleaser in you that says you will be happy once everyone else is happy. Sometimes it's just not possible to make everybody else happy, so you are delaying your own happiness for an outcome that won't be realized.

Learn that you should focus instead on satisfying somebody else: your-self. If you are asked for something, consider whether the request is feasible. Does it meet your needs? Can it bring you a sense of satisfaction as well? If so, then by all means engage. If not, say no. People-pleasing behavior is born of fear. When we act from that place, we are assuming that others are in charge. When we act from a genuine desire to be true to ourselves instead, we operate from a healthy place and exhibit the behaviors that are best for everyone.

DAY

—•— **334** —•—

Be Daring

Stepping out of my comfort zone is a great way to energize my psyche. Whether it is eating something I wouldn't normally try or speaking up in a situation where I'd normally remain quiet, I always feel a boost of confidence once I am done. Over time, I have found that we sometimes decide how we feel about something prematurely, without an open mind, or without all the information we need to consider. I think I won't like sushi, and then find that I love it. I'm convinced that going to a NASCAR race will bore me to tears, and then I wind up sitting beside a fascinating woman. Being open to new experiences—and willing to be changed by them—allows us the opportunity and room to grow. It gives our life flavor and our souls fervor.

Today —— Do something that is daring for you. It doesn't have to be major—like bungee jumping or sky diving. It just needs to be something that is out of your normal realm of possibility, something that gives you the sense that you are really living. You might go to a movie in a genre that normally doesn't appeal to you, cook a new recipe, write a sonnet, try a new cuisine. When you are done, savor the adrenaline rush or confidence boost you get from the endeavor.

— 335 —

Surround Yourself with Positive People

Have any energy suckers in your life? You know the type. Energy suckers are the people who ask too much of you over and over again, aren't afraid to put you out or put you down, take pleasure in your pain, and take pain in your pleasure. Let me guess, you've kept them around because you haven't wanted to hurt their feelings, even though they hurt your feelings over and over and over again. Energy suckers keep us from being our best selves because we are too busy tending to them or licking our wounds from them. By spending so much time with those who are negative, we begin to dwell in the negative ourselves, which isn't good for our sense of well-being or confidence.

Today ——— Choose to surround yourself with positive people. This doesn't mean you have to break up with the more negative people in your life right now (although you may choose to do this). It simply means you are distributing time and energy in a way that will nurture and support you and the healthy relationships you have.

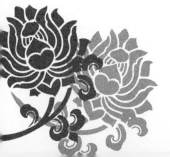

— 336 —

Watch *Good Hair*

I was walking down the hall of my high school with a friend who was African American.

"How was your weekend?" I asked.

"Fine," she said. "I got my hair permed. Did some homework. Hung out."

I looked at her hair. It wasn't curly.

"Your hair's not curly."

Tiffany could tell I was totally confused. "Perms on black people don't make their hair curly, Rosie. Perms make our hair straight."

Years later, I would watch my African American girlfriends in college go through it with their hair. And, now, with an African son, we are even more privy to black hair culture.

"Oh, your baby has that good hair," the women on my street will tell me.

Hair. We talk about good hair and bad hair. We talk about good hair days and bad hair days. It can affect our body image. It can affect our sense of self. We could be beautiful if only . . . our hair were straight, curly, longer, shorter, thicker, thinner, blonder, darker.

Today — Rent and watch *Good Hair*. This documentary by Chris Rock takes a look at black hair culture and was inspired by his daughter, who asked him why she didn't have good hair. While some of us might think, "But it's not about me," what it shows about our hang-ups and the lengths we go to for beauty is universally revealing.

— 337 —

Have a Musical Meditation

W e've looked at various ways to meditate over the course of this year. Today we are experiencing another option.

Today — Select an album or a playlist you have created that signifies reflection to you. Lay down somewhere and listen to it. Just listen, letting your thoughts go wherever the music takes you.

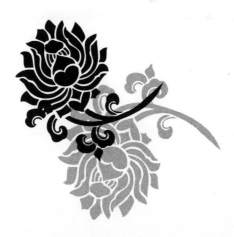

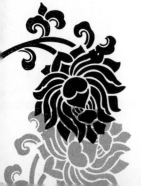

— 338 —

Break Into Blossom

I n the poem, *A Blessing*, James Wright writes:

Suddenly, I realize
That if I stepped out of my body I would
Break into blossom.

Today ⟶ Consider the simplicity and power of this sentence: *If I stepped out of my body, I would break into blossom.* Indeed, being consumed by our bodies is a guaranteed way to weigh ourselves down in this world, to keep ourselves from realizing our best selves. Body worries are a distracting force, a force that takes away from our power, our truth, our ability, our passion. Realize, instead, that beauty comes from opening up, like a flower. Allow yourself, today, to go out and break into blossom.

—■ 339 ■—

Talk Less

Sometimes we fill the air with so many of our thoughts, so many incomplete ideas and stories, that we forget to take things in, to breathe, to learn, to listen.

Today ⟶ Quit spinning your tales and just listen, do, and be today. Talk less than you normally would and see what lessons come to you in the silence.

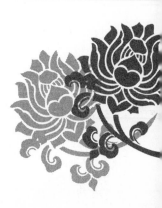

— 340 —

Form a Brain Trust

Having people we can go to for advice is so helpful, but sometimes we hesitate asking questions of them. A few years ago, when Circle de Luz was just a nugget of an idea in my mind, I was helped tremendously by the insight of friends whose brains I picked while we were working out, eating lunch, or having a meeting. When I took my idea to several focus groups, I got even more feedback, and the project moved forward. Asking people to share their insight, I realized, is one of the surest ways to move in the direction of our dreams with confidence.

Today —— Form a brain trust. Invite three to four other people to join you for dinner, ice cream, or coffee. These people don't necessarily have to know each other. Each person should come to the "date" with a question that has been on his or her mind—a problem that needs some solving. Give everyone the opportunity to ask their questions, then give each person in the group an opportunity to problem solve and voice some solutions. The point is not to *discuss* the situation. It is simply to provide the questioner with new ways of addressing the issue. After your meeting, go to a quiet place and reflect on the suggestions you received about your situation. Write about them in your *Beautiful You* journal and follow your thoughts through to their conclusion.

Write a Mission Statement

Mission statements allow you to voice what you want for yourself, how you want to be in the world, what matters to you, and your dreams. Mission statements are a powerful part of self-empowerment.

When I had my students write mission statements, I used Stephen Covey's approach, made popular in *The Seven Habits of Highly Effective People,* for developing a principle-centered mission statement. Students would list their values, the roles they played in life, how they wanted to be seen in each role, and the dreams they had for themselves and their lives. They would then read over what they wrote, looking for repetitive or similar themes—recurring notions that would help shape their mission statements. When it came time to write the statements, I encouraged them to do it in a form that resonated with them.

When I was 25, my mission statement was a list of declarative sentences. But after I learned more about myself and my purpose in life, my mission statement grew more streamlined. At 35, I summarized my mission in one complex sentence, a method I learned from Nicole Greer, a life coach who is part of the national training team for Laurie Beth Jones's *The Path: Creating Your Mission Statement for Work and for Life.*

"A mission statement really gets at the soul of what we are doing and what we really want to be about," Greer explains. "We want to consciously think about it and have it become part of our fiber."

Jones's formula for writing a one-sentence mission statement has three parts.

"It needs to have a core value. Something that you know is most important to you. Next, you need to think about the things you innately do and describe it with three verbs. Finally, you have to identify who you are most meant to serve in this world," says Greer, whose own mission is "to energize, impact, and influence people to lead vibrant lives through engaging the possibilities."

My mission statement after meeting with Greer?

"Rosie Molinary specializes in encouraging individuals to explore, integrate, and solidify their voices in order to empower them with their own truth, confidence, hope, passion, and action."

Today ⟶ Write a mission statement for both the life you are living and the life you most want to live. The one-sentence method is easy to memorize and serves as a sound-bite-size reminder whenever you need it. Sometimes, though, you need a comprehensive list. Ultimately, it is important for your mission statement to be positive and to serve as a guide in your daily life, a compass that helps ensure you are always moving toward your own true north.

⋯ 342 ⋯

Save for a Rainy Day

There is the deliberate savings you do each month when you deposit money into your savings account (make sure this is happening after your budget overhaul!). And then there is the satisfaction of watching a piggy bank or coin jar fill up right in front of you. One of my friends has a family member who keeps a large water jug on display and drops a five dollar bill inside whenever one lands in her pocket. As a girl, I had a piggy bank that I put all my dimes—and only dimes—in. Now, we save all of our pocket change daily. At the end of the month, we exchange it for dollars to put in our son's piggy bank.

Today ⋯ Pick a vessel and a strategy and start saving at home. Having a container in which you stash extra cash provides a visual reminder that you have taken your security into your own hands. Your empowerment ultimately leads to greater confidence.

— 343 —

Work a Room

For years, I could find myself in most any situation and feel comfortable. But after I left the education field and began writing fulltime, I found that I was significantly more shy. I always knew that I was an introvert—even when I taught and coached and had to be "on" 14 hours a day. But my introversion soared to a whole new level once I started working from home. Now, I often feel shy and unsure of myself when I show up at a place where chatting people up—much less charming them—is required, especially if I am not there for work. Losing that confidence that used to come so naturally to me has been a revelation. I thought that confidence was innate to me. What I have learned is that it came from practice. With that insight, I have been trying to reengage the courage and fearlessness I used to feel in abundance by practicing deliberately engaging in conversation.

Today —— Work a room. Engaging with other people means finding common ground and showing interest. Maybe you admire a piece of jewelry the woman next to you is wearing or are curious about how you are both connected to the event. Maybe you are curious about her work or her hobbies. Don't be too afraid to ask questions—and don't worry that your questions aren't smart. Sometimes the smartest questions are the ones that ask someone to start at the very beginning. What I have learned as a writer is that people love being asked about their stories. Look the person you are speaking to in the eye, and nod to show her you are paying attention. Don't be afraid to make connections based on things you have seen or read. And if the conversation isn't as dynamic as you'd hoped, don't take it personally. It takes two people to make a conversation sing. Instead, let the person know it was a pleasure and move on. With practice, you'll see that you can build a conversation by establishing connections as entry points, and you'll begin to feel more and more confident.

— 344 —

Read *Clorinda* to a Child in Your Life

One of the sweetest gifts given to our baby boy was the book *Clorinda*. Written by Robert Kinerk, it follows the story of a spunky cow who dreams of becoming a ballerina. My sweet friend Anna inscribed the following inside the front cover: "Follow your dreams, sweet baby, and always know you are everything warm, bright, loving, and strong to all who are so grateful to love you so." It is the most perfect of messages for our baby, and it matches the message of *Clorinda,* too.

Today —— Stop by your local library or bookstore and pick up *Clorinda*. Then read and discuss this charming tale with a little boy or little girl in your life. Talk about the importance of dreams, about whether or not Clorinda's journey was a success, and about what lesson the little one in your life can take away from this wonderful book.

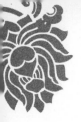

Attend a Lecture

When I was in my early twenties, I heard Maya Angelou speak. She was as thrilling as you might imagine, her deep rasp of a voice expounding wisdom at the rate of one brilliant thought per minute. I was on the cusp of starting my teaching career, so when she said, "When the student is ready, the teacher appears," something lit up within me. I wanted to be the student who declared herself ready and then knew to keep an eye out for the teacher—whether or not that teacher was a person or an experience. I wanted, too, to be the teacher wise enough to notice when I was being beckoned to help facilitate the lesson that one of my students most needed at that moment, even if it had nothing to do with United States History (the subject I taught most).

A few years later, when I was teaching, I heard Gloria Steinem speak. The auditorium was packed, and as she began, a small infant began to weep. The mother couldn't silence him, so she tried to discretely sneak out of the auditorium, hoping, I am sure, not to bother the other audience members.

"Don't go," Steinem said, interrupting her remarks. "We put up with so much noise in our lives—beepers and cell phones, sirens and car alarms. The least any of us can do is be patient with the sounds of a child." That remark has stayed with me so many years later. I was impressed by Steinem's acknowledgment of the child's voice, the humanity she exhibited in noting his humanity, and the way she cut away from her prepared remarks to teach all of us a quiet and powerful lesson.

Going to lectures throughout my life has been such a valuable education. There is always something that sticks with me, informing my sensibilities, long after the night has passed. I become a better person just by spending an evening with someone who has so much to share.

Today ⟶ Scan the calendar pages of colleges and universities near you, or check out the literary calendar in your local newspaper. Choose something that interests you and put that upcoming lecture on your calendar.

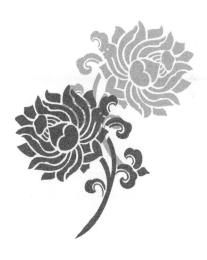

—•• 346 ••—

Finish These Sentences

On Day 42, you finished these sentences. Today, we are revisiting them.

Today —— In your *Beautiful You* journal, finish these sentences. Then, compare them to your answers on Day 42.

I can...
I will...
I expect...
I look forward to...
I hope...
I wish...
I plan...

— 347 —

Drop Everything and Read

Sometimes it is helpful to just get out of our own heads for awhile, and one of the best ways to do that is to read. Research from the Mind Lab at the University of Sussex has revealed that reading for as little as ten minutes can lower one's heart rate and reduce stress. When we feel less stressed, we feel more comfortable in our skin.

Today —— Email or phone people whose reading tastes might lead you to a fabulous find and ask them what they recommend. Jot down all their suggestions and then go to a book store, library, or audiobook vendor and select one of them to read or listen to for at least 10 minutes today. For just that time, escape from yourself and your own preoccupations and enjoy your read.

—• 348 •—

Get Trained as a Dove Self-Esteem Fund Facilitator

As a part of the Dove Campaign for Real Beauty, the Dove Self-Esteem Fund helps girls build positive self-esteem and body image. Dove invites women around the world to sign up for a CD-based training program that will prepare them to facilitate body-image and self-image workshops for girls.

Today —• Are you feeling particularly compelled to continue this work in a deliberate way? Visit www.dove.us and learn more about the Self-Esteem Fund's efforts. Sign up to be a Dove Self-Esteem Fund program facilitator and you'll soon receive training materials in the mail; you'll learn everything you need to host a workshop for girls in your community.

— 349 —

Go Horseback Riding

Horseback riding is such a sensational experience. As your horse swiftly moves, you feel the wind in your hair. The lushness of your horse's mane and coat is a pleasure between your fingers. Your senses are on alert as you try to synchronize your movements with your horse's movements; the muscles in your arms, legs, and core channel a kind of electricity as you ride. When you are horseback riding, you can't help but feel vital and present. It's a wonderful way to practice how we should engage life.

Today — Go horseback riding. Visit the websites of some of your local parks to see if they offer horseback riding on site, or enter "horseback riding" and the name of your city in your favorite Internet search engine.

—→ 350 ←—

Consider Your Own Advice

We all know so much more than we give ourselves credit for knowing. We often dispense useful advice to others that we don't always heed ourselves. By tapping into what we already know deep within, we allow ourselves greater access to our own truth.

Today ——→ In your *Beautiful You* journal, record what advice you would give a niece, coworker, friend, or daughter about life, self-awareness, self-esteem, self-care, and body image.

Tell a Girl She is Fabulous

After *Hijas Americanas* came out, a sixth-grade teacher invited me to come speak to her Latina students, and I gladly accepted the invitation. I have been visiting with these girls for the past several years.

At that first meeting, I asked the girls about their dreams. All of them planned on graduating from high school and continuing their education. They were sweet and earnest, and I couldn't help but fall in love with them. I kept going back. I believe in and want the best for them, and I want them to know how precious they are.

One Saturday, when the girls were in eighth grade, their sixth-grade teacher and I took them out to lunch. We all started pouring over the menu, figuring out what we would have. And then Mia, one of these lovely girls, said something that stole my breath away.

"I'm on a diet."

Her former teacher and I both pounced, telling her empathetically that she was perfect the way she was, that she didn't need to be on a diet, etc. My heart just hurt over it until I saw her order a perfectly normal meal and exhibit a perfectly normal appetite. After that, it hurt just a smidge less, but I still worried about what she had said.

Meanwhile, we talked about school, about how the girls liked eighth grade. Mia, who had been a bit of an underachiever in the sixth and seventh grades and was often in trouble, said, "I think I am smarter than I used to be. Before, I never thought I could do the homework so I would just copy someone else's. Now I know I can do the homework and so I just do it all myself."

We talked about growing older and more confident, about doubting yourself when you shouldn't, about the joy of trusting your own ability. Later, I marveled at how well these girls were growing up, despite the odds against them—some of which they actually create for themselves. I want so much for them to be safe, happy, confident, and focused. I want so much for them to love themselves, to be fully possessed of themselves. I want so much for the steps that take them backwards to stop, for the steps that move them forward to quicken. I want them to have just one moment to see themselves through my eyes.

I can't guarantee that any of that will happen, but I can guarantee that I will always show up for them, that I will challenge and toast them, that I will journey with them anywhere.

Today ⟶ Engage in a genuine, deep conversation with a girl in your life. Share what you know, what you are still learning, and what you admire about her.

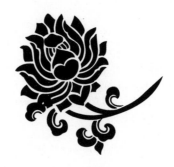

Make a List

Earlier this year, we practiced taking more sensory pleasure in our lives. Today we're assessing how well we are doing at finding the divine and pleasurable in more of our experiences.

Today —— In your *Beautiful You* journal, write a list of five things you love to touch, five things you love to taste, five things you love to see, five things you love to smell, and five things you love to hear.

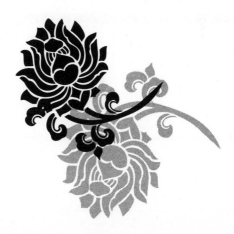

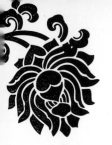

— 353 —

Try a Team Sport

As I mentioned earlier, I traveled to Brazil in my mid-twenties with ten students and a co-leader. We were there to help build a pediatric medical clinic, drill wells, and build latrines for a community in the rain forest. While we worked every day, nights found us playing soccer with kids, each other, and the masons we worked with during the day. It had been years since I had played on a team (many, many, many years), and I was worried that I would bring the team down. What I found instead was that I loved it—and that no one paid attention to any of my self-perceived flaws. We simply enjoyed each other and the game while learning skills that helped us in our daily work—how to function as a team, how to adapt to different personalities, when to ask for help, when to be supportive, when to go for it on our own. With each game, I grew more and more confident and the members of our team grew more and more adept at working with each other.

Today —— Try a team sport. You don't have to join an ultracompetitive league; maybe all you have the time for is a recreational kickball game or a doubles tennis match with some friends. Just squeeze whatever game you can into your schedule so you can reap the benefits of the experience.

— 354 —

Make a "Wish Jar"

To help our aspirations and hopes come true, it is helpful to name them and put them out into the universe. By truly making our desires known, at least to ourselves, we pay more attention to them and begin to gather the information and resolve we need to realize them.

Today ——— Clean out an old jar and create a new label for it that represents you. Gather scraps of decorative paper and keep them nearby. Periodically, jot down a note about something you're dreaming about or hoping to have in your life; when you're done, put the note in the jar. A new job? A new mindset? New sheets? New shoes? World peace? Inner peace? It's your wish jar. Anything goes.

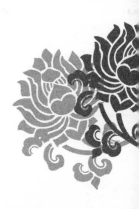

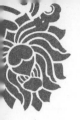

Tune in to "This I Believe"

A couple of years ago, I immersed myself in reading *This I Believe*. It's a collection of short essays inspired by the National Public Radio series of the same name, in which Americans from all walks of life—famous and not so famous—read an essay that completes the thought begun in the book's title. In each essay, the author writes about the one thing he or she believes in and why, in just a few hundred words. The essays are very brief capsules of a life that uniquely capture the essence of who we are.

I have taught workshops where participants go through exercises that ultimately lead them to their belief statements. The statements people shared were always remarkable—so much so that I still remember many of them:

I believe in the power of a Christmas carol.

I believe in the backyard garden.

This I believe... Nerds Rule.

I believe in the power of the underdog.

I believe in listening.

Listening to other people's beliefs is powerful for me; it helps me see my own life differently and more deliberately. When we begin to consistently see our lives through a deliberate lens, one etched in values, the grip of impossible beauty standards loosens. And when the grip loosens, we begin to live a life of our imagining, rooted in what is real.

Today — Go to NPR's website, www.npr.org, and listen to at least five "This I Believe" recordings.

— 356 —

Write Your Own "This I Believe" Statement

In preparing to teach my "This I Believe" Statement workshop, I toyed around with many of my own beliefs, reducing each to a one-sentence sound bite that might later lead to a longer individual belief statement.

Here is part of the list that I brainstormed:

I believe in the power of voice.

I believe that exposure changes everything.

I believe that a little cupcake goes a long way.

I believe that our passion is our purpose.

I believe that powerful learning happens with an emotional connection.

I believe that even when you don't know what to say, you show up.

But this was the unedited statement I ultimately ended up writing:

When my best friend's father died, I rushed to her side on her family's Mississippi farm. As it has always done, seeing my dear friend and her family filled my well. But grieving the impossible loss of my friend's father, a man who so many respected and loved, is the kind of thing that will split you open. When we left the church, the procession streamed out onto the Mississippi streets, winding miles and miles out to farmland, and I was reminded about a beautiful custom that still happens in some smaller Southern towns. Every car on the street pulled over and stopped for the duration of this miles-long processional. People on the sidewalks took off their hats, covered their hearts. No one looked impatient. Not one person was on a cell phone as I drove by. They were people of all ages, all cultures, stopped. I wondered for a moment if I would have known at 16 to pull over and show this amount of respect—the way I saw one shirtless teenage boy do in his pickup truck. For miles, we drove by stopped car after stopped car. After having spent the entire day before with the dozens and dozens of family members who were tenderly holding each other in so much love, after watching a visitation line wind through the church with people who waited three hours to tell the family what this man had meant to them, after one of the most lovely celebrations of life; after all of this, riding down that long road with every car pulled over, every walking person halted, every police officer stopping traffic with his hand over his heart, I was so very humbled by the magnitude of what his life meant and also by the magnitude of what every one of our lives really means. In that spirit, I add the most true statement to my list: I believe that every life is worth stopping for.

Today ⟶ Write your own *This I Believe* statement in your *Beautiful You* journal. It doesn't need to be perfect or long. It simply needs to capture something you know to be true, something that guides you at your core and shows you that you are more than your looks and your body.

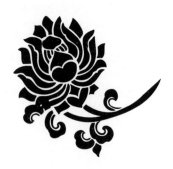

— 357 —

Join a Group

When I left my job as a college administrator to write full-time, I didn't anticipate how my new working environment—all alone in my home—might affect my confidence and sense of self. Before my new career, many of my strengths were related to being in communion with people. Without that, I naturally lost some of my confidence. What worked for me in trying to reestablish my sense of self was deliberately coming together with others—whether at a book club or as a member of a nonprofit board. By being with others, I could connect, share my experiences, learn from others, and get outside of the smaller vacuum of my world.

Today —— Consider joining—or forming—a group. Been thinking that it would be nice to discuss books with other readers? Ask around to see if there is a book club you could join, or form your own. Love knitting? Join a knitting circle at your local yarn store. Have another interest that you want to develop? Look for groups that make sense—like triathlon training groups or writing circles—and sign up. By branching out socially and developing your interests, you nurture yourself and build confidence.

— 358 —

Consider Your Inspiration

You have spent almost a year considering yourself, your life, and the world around you. Hopefully, you have been moved and lifted by what you have thought about and experienced. Those moments can serve as inspiration for you as you move forward.

Today —— In your *Beautiful You* journal, answer these questions: What inspires you? What makes you feel a sense of awe?

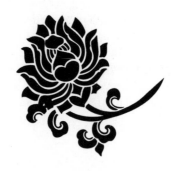

— 359 —

Sprout Something

When we lack confidence, we can easily feel defeated and remove ourselves from situations and experiences too early or too easily. Sometimes the best way to build our confidence is to allow ourselves to be inspired by someone else in an area where that person excels. The point is not to compare ourselves to someone else but to allow ourselves to truly feel or see someone else's gift—and to be inspired by it.

Today — Visit an art exhibit and select one piece of artwork that speaks to you, or pick up a book of poetry and select one poem that touches you in some way. Using that piece as your inspiration, create your own work of art or poem. Rather than comparing your work to the original, consider how being open to appreciating the original allowed you to create this new work. By being open to what is before us, we can challenge ourselves and grow in new ways that allow us to blossom.

Sign Up for Sewing Classes

In *Love is a Mix Tape*, Rob Sheffield reflects on how Renee, his curvy wife, began to make her own clothes, leading her to real empowerment. Sheffield writes:

> The more she sewed, the easier it got for her to move and breathe, since she now had clothes she could move and breathe in, and feel totally hot while she did so.... Renee's sewing was a way for her to follow the changes in her body. She felt her hips growing more and more Appalachian, marking her as one of her people.... There was a lot of history in the hips, and Renee was learning her history. With that sewing machine, she was making history of her own.

I read this passage and immediately marked it. Both for Renee's power and presence and ability to champion her self, but also for Rob's ability to see it, appreciate it, and celebrate it. Renee's sewing reminds me of the only times that I feel sad about the way my body is changing as I grow older. Those times usually occur in a dressing room, when I realize that yet another designer just doesn't understand breasts and hips (and doesn't understand that women with breasts and hips really want fabulous clothes too). In recent years, I've learned not to covet the styles I used to love, but sometimes I just can't help it. Wouldn't it be much more empowering if I learned how to sew instead, so that I could re-create the styles with my own body in mind?

Today — If this idea strikes you, check out the continuing education opportunities in your area and sign up for a sewing class. When you're not forced to depend on other people to make clothes that perfectly fit your body, you feel a greater sense of liberation.

— 361 —

Have a Child Draw Another Picture

As you may recall, on Day 15 you asked a child to draw a self-portrait. Over the past eleven months, you have been working on your own self-care, self-awareness, and self-esteem issues while also nurturing this child's developing sense of self.

Today —— Have the child draw another self-portrait, then pull out the old self-portrait and look it over with the child. What has changed? What has stayed the same? Why is that?

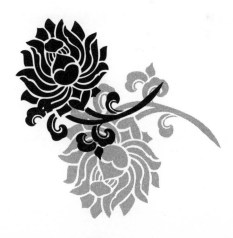

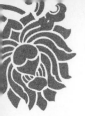

— 362 —

Draw Another Picture of Yourself

On Day 16, you drew a self-portrait. Since then, you have been actively engaged in addressing issues of self-esteem, self-awareness, and body image. How you perceive yourself now is likely different from how you once did.

Today —— Draw a self-portrait. Now compare it to your last self-portrait. In your *Beautiful You* journal, reflect on what has changed. Why is that? What is still the same? Why is that? What do you wish to see in a future self-portrait?

— 363 —

Consider This Call to Action

In *Hijas Americanas*, I wrote a call to action that began with these words:

All of us—regardless of what we suffered through because of our breasts, our hair, our noses, our skin, our family, our finances, our accents, our attributes—still have had so much entrusted to us. Our ancestors, grandparents, or parents bravely navigated a new land in the name of their futures and the futures of their offspring; in so doing, they paved the way for the lives that we're living. We have the option to take that hope and stretch further, reach higher, do more. The body and beauty revolution is ours to begin. It's time to give ourselves, and the girls and women around us, a wider lens through which to consider our beauty and who we are beyond our beauty. We have to bite our tongues when a moment of self-loathing or criticism enters our minds. We have to encourage the women we love to talk about something other than their cellulite. We have to eradicate these limiting thoughts from our minds, because a change in our own minds leads to change in our media and on our planet. On your bad days, call someone who loves you as you are, and bask in the respect they give you. If you don't have someone like that in your life, perhaps you need to examine why and start looking.

The expectations we absorb can either encourage us or limit us. They can catapult us to possibility or keep us confined by our feelings of inadequacy. There is an old saying that tells us we are only as strong as our weakest link, and it's true in this case. Body image isn't just the problem of the insecure girl. Having confidence does not mean that body-image issues will not affect you. If your child's teacher is plagued by low self-esteem, it affects how she champions your child; it affects you. The way women have been reduced in our world affects all of us, directly and indirectly. If the women of the next generation are crippled by their lack of confidence, their leader-ship will falter, and their ability to make change will be compromised.

Today —— Consider what these words mean to you. Write about it in your *Beautiful You* journal.

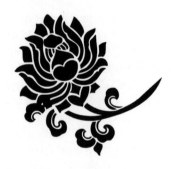

— 364 —

Champion All Women

The passage continues:

Champion all women. We need to know that as long as one
woman is crippled by feelings of inadequacy, then the world that we
have created is inadequate. Supporting one another and freeing one
another from the limiting messages that we internalize can be revo-
lutionary. We make the choice whether to internalize these messages.
We make the choice whether to build up or tear down. We can have
power in our lives by not taking in negative messages, and we can
empower other women by not sending out negative messages.

We are all beautiful and powerful women, and we must make the
choice to always present our authentic selves. Don't box others in;
don't relegate someone to a space she hasn't chosen for herself. . . .

When we begin to see women in all of their dimensions, we begin to
eradicate confining stereotypes and worldviews. We start to see...all
women as complex individuals, and not just as part of a larger stereo-
typical whole. Look wider, acknowledge more, think bigger. We are
women of all colors and cultures, and we can make a world that does
not relegate us to type and cast. We can choose to live in a world that
celebrates wholeness and complexities in our women. We can choose
to create a society that encourages women to be healthier and more
whole, a society that unites us in our commonalities while acknowledging the depth of the individual. The more we challenge the limits
we place on each other, the more open the world will be to all of us.

Today — Raise your voice and demand an end to a narrowly defined
beauty mystique. No matter where you have been on the journey to self-
hood, start each day with the intention of championing yourself and others. It is never too late to claim yourself, to celebrate your own brilliance
and the brilliance of all women.

Celebrate Your Brilliance

A year ago, you began this journey. You wanted to enhance your self-awareness, embrace your sense of self, and celebrate your brilliance in order to be able to engage more deliberately in the world, in your world. Over the course of the last twelve months, you have vigorously done the work to arrive at a place where you could be released from the consuming consideration of yourself, so that you might engage in the work of your life. Congratulations!

Today —— First, celebrate the journey you have just taken in a way that has meaning to you. Next, consider where things stand today. In your *Beautiful You* journal, describe what you have discovered about yourself over the past year. How have you grown? What do you appreciate about this journey? What is your brilliance? How will you continue to recognize it and offer it to the world?

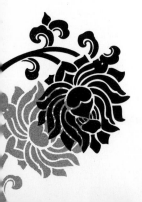

Notes

Day 6   Tucker, K., Martz, D., Curtin, L., and Bazzini, D. "Examining 'Fat Talk' experimentally in a female dyad: How are women influenced by another woman's body presentational style?" *Body Image: An International Journal of Research 4* (2007): 157-174.

Day 11   Molinary, Rosie. "The Latina in Me." *Waking Up American: Coming of Age Biculturally,* ed. Angela Jane Founty (Berkeley: Seal Press, 2005).

Day 59   Fea, Courtney. "Effect of Trait Self-Objectification on Body Shame, Appearance Anxiety and Unipolar Depression". *American Psychological Society's Annual Convention.* (2005).

Day 60   Want, S.C., Vickers, K., and Amos, J. "The influence of television programs on appearance satisfaction: Making and mitigating social comparisons to *Friends*. *Sex Role*s 60 (2009): 642-655.

Day 66   Campbell, A., and Hausenblas, H. A. "Effects of exercise interventions on body image: A meta-analysis." *Journal of Health Psychology* 14 (2009): 780-793

Day 85   Hart, S., Field, T., Hernandez-Reif, M., Nearing, G., Shaw, S., Schanberg, S., and Kuhn, C. "Anorexia nervosa symptoms are reduced by massage therapy." *Eating Disorders* 9 (2001): 289-99.

Day 96   Niemiec, C., Ryan, R., and Deci, E. "The path taken: Consequences of attaining intrinsic and extrinsic aspirations in college life." *Journal of Research in Personality* 3 (2009): 291-206.

Day 117   Molinary, Rosie. "Why Do We Stay?" *Skirt! Magazine*, October 2008.

Day 228   Etcoff, N., Orbach, S., Scott, J., and D'Agostino, H. "Beyond Stereotypes: Rebuilding the Foundation of Beauty Beliefs: Findings of the 2005 Global Study." Dove, Unilever PLC, 2006.

Day 264   Pipher, Mary. *Seeking Peace: Chronicles of the Worst Buddhist in the World* (New York: Riverhead Books, 2009), 169.

Day 265   Stone, Judith. "This is What Happy Looks Like." *Good Housekeeping*, September 2009, 195.

Day 278   Daubenmier, Jennifer. "The relationship of yoga, body awareness, and body responsiveness to self-objectification and disordered eating." *Psychology of Women Quarterly* 29 (2005): 207-219.

Day 300   Dunn, E.W., Aknin, L., and Norton, M.I. "Spending money on others promotes happiness." *Science* 319 (2008): 1687-1688.

Day 360   Sheffield, Rob. *Love is a Mix Tape: Life and Loss, One Song at a Time* (New York: Three Rivers Press, 2007), 114-115.

Day 363   Molinary, Rosie. *Hijas Americanas: Beauty, Body Image, and Growing Up Latina* (Berkeley: Seal Press, 2007), 276-277.

Day 364   Ibid.

Acknowledgments

I am indebted to so many people who helped to make this book, this journey, real.

The women of *Hijas Americanas: Beauty, Body Image, and Growing Up Latina*, the women I met around the country as I was promoting the book, and my students all sensitized me to the urgency of this work. I am humbled to have heard their stories and to have been able to witness some of their experiences, and I am grateful for the inspiration that they have each provided me.

A conversation with gifted writer Jodi Helmer led me to the concept behind this book, and further conversations with and guidance from Erin Lane Beam led to the book's heart.

Thank you to Brooke Warner at Seal Press for seeing the worth of this book and to Krista Lyons for shepherding it into creation.

Everyone at Seal Press is a class act. I am honored and humbled to be in their company and to benefit from their many gifts.

Thank you to Erin Lane Beam, Laura Caputo, Harriet Kessler, Jenny Kinney, Isha Ahsan Lee, Julie McCue, Jill Williams, and Marguerite Williams for your generosity as first readers. Because of the generosity you exhibited and your smart, helpful, honest insight, *Beautiful You* is a better work.

Molly Barker, Dr. Amy Combs, and Julie Hall are each an inspiration to me.

The work that they do is urgent, inspired, and transformative, and I am grateful to learn at their feet every day. Dr. Combs graciously answered questions and discussed issues with me throughout the research and writing process. Her expertise and kindness are so appreciated.

My husband and son kept me company on the long days of editing and organizing, kept me humbled by rearranging my stacks, and kept me sane by reminding me that we recognize our beauty and celebrate our brilliance when we choose to immerse ourselves in each other and the worth and work of this world. You are both so immensely loved.

Every Friday morning, I walk into a classroom and share the experience of life and this journey toward brilliance with compelling students. That I have the incredible good fortune to engage with them in this journey humbles me. That I have the opportunity to learn from them inspires me. That we have the capacity to change the world because of our dialogue and the action it generates thrills me.

This is our world, these are our choices, and this is our chance.

Let's all change the conversation so we can change the consequence.

About the Author

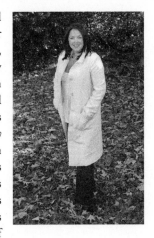

An author, speaker, teacher, and activist, Rosie Molinary had earlier careers as a high school teacher, coach, and college administrator. Her poetry and nonfiction have been published in various literary magazines and books, and she has contributed to various magazines and websites. *Hijas Americanas: Beauty, Body Image, and Growing Up Latina*, her book on the coming-of-age experiences of Latinas in America, was published by Seal Press in 2007. In addition to writing, she teaches a course on body image for the women's studies department at the University of North Carolina at Charlotte and speaks around the country on body image, diversity, self-awareness, social justice, and writing.

Raised in Columbia, South Carolina, she graduated from Davidson College with a degree in African American studies and certification as a high school social studies teacher. She earned her Masters in Fine Arts in creative writing at Goddard College.

In her free time, Rosie works on various social justice issues. She also paints, runs, and obsesses over NFL football and her fantasy football team. She currently serves as the board chairman for Circle de Luz, a nonprofit program that provides mentoring, programming, and scholarship support to young Latinas. Rosie lives with her husband and son in North Carolina.

Selected Titles from Seal Press

For more than thirty years, Seal Press has published
groundbreaking books. By women. For women.

Hijas Americanas: Beauty, Body Image, and Growing Up Latina, by Rosie
Molinary. $15.95, 978-1-58005-189-7. Molinary highlights the nuances, complexities, and challenges of Latina femininity, sexuality, beauty and body image.

Girls' Studies: Seal Studies, by Elline Lipkin. $14.95, 978-1-58005-248-1. A look
at the socialization of girls in today's society and the media's influence on gender norms, expectations, and body image.

The Purity Myth: How America's Obsession with Virginity Is Hurting Young Women,
by Jessica Valenti. $16.95, 1-58005-314-3. Valenti presents a powerful argument
that girls and women, even in this day and age, are overly valued for their sexuality—and that this needs to stop.

Body Outlaws: Rewriting the Rules of Beauty and Body Image, edited by Ophira
Edut, foreword by Rebecca Walker. $15.95, 978-1-58005-108-8. Filled with honesty and humor, this groundbreaking anthology offers stories by women who
have chosen to ignore, subvert, or redefine the dominant beauty standard in
order to feel at home in their bodies.

Living Canvas: Your Total Guide to Tattoos, Piercings, and Body Modification, by
Karen L. Hudson. $17.95, 978-1-58005-288-7. A helpful resource for body art
enthusiasts, whether you're thinking about getting your first or fifth tattoo,
planning for your next bod-mod, or regretting a negative experience.

Find Seal Press Online
www.SealPress.com
www.Facebook.com/SealPress
Twitter: @SealPress